Testimonials

In a convincing, easy to follow way, Dr. Somborac shows the causes of the shocking rise in excess weight, diabetes, heart disease and other "diseases of civilization", how dental decay forecasts them and how to prevent them. As Hippocrates taught us, health is the greatest human blessing. I highly recommend this book.

Gordon Nikiforuk, DDS, MSc, FRCD, FCID, Professor and Dean Emeritus, Faculty of Dentistry, University of Toronto

---

This is a must read. It is intellectually provocative and ultimately a compelling view of opportunities missed by oral health professionals. However, its message is prudently and sensibly articulated so as to reassure us that a less technologically linear and more disciplined approach to avoiding disease patterns is indeed feasible.

George A. Zarb, B.Ch.D., D.D.S., M.S. (Mich.), M.S. (Ohio State), F.R.C.D. (C), Professor Emeritus, Faculty of Dentistry, University of Toronto

---

In this book, Dr. Somborac has stimulated all of us to look closely at a much broader scope for our professional responsibilities. We dentists see patients on a much more frequent basis than others in health care. He has opened our eyes to the possibility to help others with their overall health while we accomplish our specialized portion of healthcare.

Gordon J. Christensen, DDS MSD, PhD, Director, Practical Clinical Courses, Diplomate, American Board of Prosthodontics, Cofounder and Senior Consultant, CR Foundation, Adjunct Professor, Brigham Young University and University of Utah

Dr. Somborac's writing is lucid. Reading *Your Mouth, Your Health* is like seeing contemporary dental and health issues through X-ray glasses.

Dr. Ansgar Cheng, Adjunct Associate Professor, National University of Singapore, Examiner, Royal College of Dentists, Canada, Prosthodontist, Special Dental Group, Singapore

---

Reading the hard science and the indisputable statistics that simple carbs are the cause of obesity, diabetes, heart disease, and more, is sobering.

Your Mouth, Your Health is a compelling and uncomplicated read that would be appropriate and life changing for all ages and education levels.

ForeWord CLARION Review (Five Stars)

In this extremely well-written book Dr. Somborac shows how profit-driven manufactured foods lead to disastrous results. Speaking as a dentist, he shows the close ties between oral disease and systemic disease. As an Italian, I'm happy to note his focus on the benefits of the Mediterranean diet. This thought-provoking book is an absolute must for everyone.

Prof. Adriano Piattelli, MD, DDS, Professor of Oral Pathology and Medicine, Dental School, University of Chieti-Pescara, Italy

YOUR MOUTH, YOUR HEALTH

YOUR MOUTH, YOUR HEALTH

Stop and Reverse Aging

MILAN SOMBORAC, DDS

iUniverse, Inc.
New York   Bloomington

Your Mouth, Your Health
Stop and Reverse Aging

You should not undertake any diet/exercise regimen recommended in this book before consulting your personal physician. Neither the author nor the publisher shall be responsible or liable for any loss or damage allegedly arising as a consequence of your use or application of any information or suggestions contained in this book.

iUniverse books may be ordered through booksellers or by contacting:

iUniverse
1663 Liberty Drive
Bloomington, IN 47403
www.iuniverse.com
1-800-Authors (1-800-288-4677)

Because of the dynamic nature of the Internet, any Web addresses or links contained in this book may have changed since publication and may no longer be valid. The views expressed in this work are solely those of the author and do not necessarily reflect the views of the publisher, and the publisher hereby disclaims any responsibility for them.

ISBN: 978-1-4502-7206-3 (pbk)
ISBN: 978-1-4502-7207-0 (cloth)
ISBN: 978-1-4502-7208-7 (ebk)

Contact author at info@drmilan.com

Printed in the United States of America

iUniverse rev. date: 3/25/10

To the late F. Logan Stanfield, commercial pilot, electrical engineer, physician, psychoanalyst, grandson of an American slave.

CONTENTS

Acknowledgments

Isaac Newton once stated, "If I have seen further than others, it is by standing upon the shoulders of giants." Many more giants walk the earth today than did in Newton's day; they publish their findings, and the great online medical libraries make the information easily available. It is easier to write a scientifically documented book today than ever before. I am deeply indebted to the clinicians and scientists who labor to coax the next nugget of truth from Mother Nature and then share it with the rest of us.

My patients have been a constant source of inspiration, especially those who refuse to become victims to modern, high-pressure methods that the international giant food companies use to put increasingly more food with increasingly less nutrient value through our bodies.

In my office, I am especially grateful to Betty-June Danylchuk, Marlene DeVries, Lynn Marshall, Bev Hooper, and Terri Skelton, who have been with me for over twenty years. They took professional pressures off me to allow me to focus on this work without losing focus on patient care.

My children, Kristin, Stefan, and Natasha; their spouses, Bobby, Jenny, and Erik; my son, Serge; and my stepdaughters, Natalie and Ashley, gave me invaluable help in the more advanced aspects of computer operations. I am particularly thankful to Natalie for taking care of important minutiae—indexing, proofreading, Web site development, and on and on.

I am indebted to John Robert Colombo, Canada's most prolific author, who offered unstinting advice about navigating the esoteric and increasingly complex world of publishing, as well as offering valuable guidance in expository writing. I want to thank Daniel Kolos, Egyptologist, for helping me adjust my usual technical writing style to one more suited to the nonspecialist.

Janet Lees, journalist and editor, walked me through the long process of understanding how writing for a lay audience needs to differ from writing for a professional audience.

Tim Brown of ROI Corporation encouraged me to write this book and introduced me to Jim Ruddy, who worked closely with me editing this book. I give Jim credit for its stylistic strengths and personally accept the blame for its stylistic weaknesses.

I want to thank friends who offered useful insights and advice: George and Barbara Weider, Dan and Debbie Erichsen-Brown, Dr. James and Irene McGillivray, Dr. Eswar and Shashi Prasad.

I hope that I have given credit to all those who deserve it and have not neglected those to whom it is owed.

Finally, I want to thank my wife, Rosi, for her boundless encouragement, support, optimism, and love. I could not even imagine a better life partner.

Preface

Putting drill to teeth or scalpel to gums makes me more money than showing patients how to bypass the drill or the scalpel in the first place—a lot more. Drill-to-teeth and scalpel-to-gums services provide dentists with a handsome living. While dental treatment is normally of excellent value for patients, it is avoidable treatment much of the time.

We dentists invest a lot of money in our education, offices, and operating costs. We do this in order to treat the ravages of dental disease as well as genetic defects and disappointments. We are set up to treat these conditions. Many of us delegate teaching patients how to forgo the need for the drill or the scalpel to our highly trained staff members. Unfortunately, when our staff is engaged in educational services, we hardly break even.

The result is that many of us wind up seeing patients again and again and providing treatments for preventable conditions—a situation we don't feel good about. We deal with the resulting unease in our own unique ways.

I wrote this book to relieve my personal frustration with my inability to transfer its content to my patients on an individual basis.

Introduction:
Most Chronic Disease Is a Choice

Like all dentists, every working day, I see tooth decay and the damage it does. In its extreme presentation, decay leads to pain, infection, fever, swelling, irritability, and occasionally even death. But there is more of a health issue here than meets the eye.

> Example 1. An overweight mother brings in her ten-year-old for relief from toothache agony. Her husband has type 2 diabetes. This overweight mother is overweight for the same reason her child has a toothache. The husband has type 2 diabetes for the same reason the mother is overweight and the child has a toothache.

> Example 2. An obese, middle-aged woman facing knee replacement surgery is in the office to make an appointment for her husband, who is about to have all his teeth removed and replaced with implant-supported teeth. The cost of this treatment is equivalent to purchasing a late-model car. This obese woman has knee replacement surgery

requirements because the knee is carrying too much weight. The cost of knee replacement surgery is also equivalent to purchasing a late-model car. She needs knee replacement surgery for the same reason her husband needs the expensive dental treatment.

Example 3. A man comes in for root canal treatment. He is overweight. So is his wife; in addition, she has varicose veins. Again, both husband and wife owe their individual ailments to a single issue.

In each of these cases, healthcare providers can trace the patients' health issues back to one thing: diet.

Families come to me, from four-year-olds to grandparents. Like all dentists, I take medical histories and see the general health problems my patients have. Most are caused by eating at the same table. The overweight mother, the child with a toothache, and the husband with diabetes all eat at the same table. The obese middle-aged woman with bad knees and her husband with bad teeth eat at the same table. The overweight man requiring root canal treatment and his overweight wife with varicose veins eat at the same table.

Years ago, I began to corroborate my own clinical findings with the work of leading researchers in the field. I started to make notes and do more research, and it soon became clear that these "diseases of civilization" are connected. These "diseases" began to be a problem only after the advent of agriculture that made civilization possible (Cordain et al. 2005). They are a different manifestation of the same problem—the problem that is the way we eat. Our nutrition has departed so significantly from the way we are built to eat that we are abusing our design, and the result is disease (Eaton 2000).

All the people in the examples above are malnourished in the same way. They eat the same "engineered food" that Big Food[1] markets. The problems start with tooth decay, and two to four

1   "Big Food" is the term we use to describe the eight hundred-pound gorilla that dominates commercial food production, distribution and marketing. As long as Big Food sells legal products and is run by business people, its detrimental influence on society's health will

decades later, other lifestyle manifestations show up (Hujoel 2009). We see them as any of the following, much more sinister, disorders:

- The "deadly quartet":
    - Excess weight and obesity
    - Elevated blood fats
    - Diabetes
    - Hypertension and resulting coronary disease

- Constipation and its consequences:
    - Varicose veins
    - Varicocele
    - Hemorrhoids
    - Diverticulitis

All of these conditions are "lifestyle diseases" that start as dental decay, which can show up as early as the age of two. In other words, when it comes to our health, tooth decay is the proverbial "canary in the coalmine," warning of imminent danger and giving us the opportunity to make changes while we still can (Hujoel 2009). If we do not heed the warning, the other conditions can show up anywhere from a few years to a few decades later (Temple and Burkitt 1993). Our unique genetic makeup determines which of the diseases we will get.

Would you like to know in your teen years whether you will get type 2 diabetes forty years down the road? Or cardiovascular disease? Or any of the other chronic diseases of civilization? Knowing an ominous future can be troubling, but knowing a manageable future is empowering. This book will empower you.

Simply stated, the refining of carbohydrates is the primary cause of these diseases. Refined carbohydrates are engineered foods. This is the key concept we'll explore, although engineered fats are increasingly adding to the problem, and we'll look into that as well.

---

increase. Big Food does provide jobs and pay taxes even though much of what it does is short on socially redeeming qualities.

Traditionally, *to refine* meant *to purify* and *to improve*. When applied to carbohydrates, to refine means *to diminish* and *to worsen*.

While total carbohydrate consumption has remained fairly consistent throughout the millennia, consumption of refined carbohydrates—mainly added sugar and white flour—over the last two hundred years is unprecedented (Cleave 1974, 14). Added sugars, any ingredient thing ending in "-ose", are sugars in our foods that exceed those found in foods naturally. Between 1970 and 2005, the North American average added-sugars intake increased by 19 percent, annually and now stands at 355 calories per day. The American Heart Association recommends a fraction of that—no more than 100 calories per day for women and 150 calories per day for men (Johnson et al. 2009). The prevalence of all the diseases this book discusses shows a parallel rise. A further thought-provoking detail is that, in societies that haven't yet adopted wide-scale use of refined carbohydrates, all of these diseases are practically absent (Richards 2002).

Dentists would be largely unemployed in a hunting and gathering society. So would physicians. There are few examples of tooth decay in pre-agricultural specimens. That is, dental decay initially appeared with the advent of the first agricultural revolution some ten thousand years ago and accelerated enormously with the advent of the Industrial Revolution some two hundred years ago. The Tigris-Euphrates region and Egypt were among the world's first areas to develop agriculture and, with it, the diseases of civilization. Ancient Egyptian mummies exhibit signs of advanced dental disease as well as the other so-called diseases of civilization (Allam et al. 2009).

We nourish our bodies today in ways that don't harmonize with our bodies' design (Hujoel 2009). We live longer today because health care has learned how to manage conditions like hypertension and diabetes; but living longer does not necessarily mean living better.

Dental decay results from knowledge and behavior problems. Obesity results from knowledge and behavior problems. Lifestyle diseases result from knowledge and behavior problems.

The purpose of this book is to show the connection between dental and overall health. How you act on that knowledge is a personal choice.

This book will resonate for you if you accept four axioms:

1. We are entirely the product of our genetic makeup and environmental influences. Nothing else shapes us.
2. Our genetic makeup is entirely beyond our control (for now, anyway).
3. Our environmental influences are significantly within our control. Distinguished scientists today continue the debate over the role of nature versus nurture in the forces that shape us. Philosophers have done so for centuries. The debate is sure to continue. For our purposes, we simply need to accept that both play a role in what we become and that we can control environment to a significant degree.
4. The methods of science are the most reliable way to uncover physiologic truths. Almost all references in this book are from primary sources from peer-reviewed scientific journals. You will find no references from Big Food-sponsored publications, gossip magazines, or supermarket tabloids.

Bottom Line

1. There is a major disconnection between the way we nourish our bodies today and the way we were designed.
2. The differences between our modern and our ancestral diets are the primary cause of the chronic diseases of civilization.
3. Dental decay, the first condition to appear, is the early warning system for any of the other health issues,

including diabetes, elevated blood fats, hypertension, excess weight and obesity, and constipation, along with its consequences (varicose veins, varicocele, hemorrhoids, deep venous thrombosis, and diverticulitis). Other conditions, such as acne, kidney disease, age-related memory decline, and many others, may also be linked to dietary choices. Ongoing research is exploring the depth of this connection.

4. With the right diet, one approximating our ancestral diet, the chronic diseases of civilization are preventable, stoppable, and reversible. (See chapter 15, "The Only Guide to Eating You'll Ever Need.")

PART I

THE FUNDAMENTALS

Chapter 1.

Our Bodies: How We (and Everything Else) Are Built

Chemicals get an unfairly bad rap as strong and powerful substances that can hurt us. The fact is, everything that exists in our physical universe is made up of chemicals—from the air we breathe, the water we drink, and the food we eat to the earth itself and every living and nonliving thing on it.[2]

In 1869, the Russian scientist Dmitri Mendeleev classified the fifty or so then-known basic chemical elements into a table in accordance to their properties (Strathern 2001). Much like the twenty-six-word alphabet can spell every word in the English language and these words can be combined to create everything from a crude joke to a Shakespearean play, so some one hundred naturally occurring elements in the modern version of Mendeleev's periodic table can be brought together to produce everything from cheap swill to great wine, from the acrid smell of bleach to the sweet aroma of a rose. The wine is contained in a glass made up of chemicals, the glass sits on a table composed of chemicals, the table and the glass have been

---

2   The ancient Greeks theorized that everything that is or ever was is made of air, fire, earth, and water. Different combinations of these four produced the endless variation of things. This theory began to falter as scientists discovered real chemical elements.

scrubbed clean with bleach made of chemicals, the rose in the vase on the table is made of chemicals—and you and I who sip the wine and smell the rose are comprised of chemicals.

Just as the letters of the alphabet are organized differently within each Shakespearean play, chemicals are organized differently within each animate and inanimate object—but perhaps not as differently as you might expect. For instance, nearly 100 percent of a common type of seashell is composed of a chemical known as hydroxyapatite—the same material that makes up much of our bone, cartilage, and teeth. In fact, these seemingly disparate entities share enough elements in common that we can get a seashell to fuse to bone. Every day, orthopedic surgeons and dentists are using the principles underlying these similar compositional elements to replace worn-out hips and missing teeth (Bobbio 1973).

Building blocks that make up a human being are called proteins, fats, vitamins, minerals, and water. All are made of chemicals. In different forms, they are also in charge of the body's many functions. The chemical combinations that are our primary source of energy are called carbohydrates.

Proteins and fats can also provide energy, in addition to being our bodies' building blocks. But this energy needs to be replenished. In addition, we need to compensate for wear and tear on the building blocks. Thus, we need to bring fuel and raw material into our bodies on an ongoing basis.

Collectively, carbohydrates, proteins, fats, vitamins, minerals, and water are called nutrients. Our bodies use them up at different rates, and therefore, we need to replace them at the appropriate rates, in the proper quantities, and with healthful qualities. That's nutrition. Nutrition comes from diet—not the kind aimed at losing weight but the kind aimed at optimal health, which should be the norm. As I've noted, the final chapter of *Your Mouth, Your Health* includes a guide to healthy eating.

Weight-loss diets have deplorable long-term results. The failure rate is virtually 100 percent! The reason is that weight-loss diets have a beginning and an end. On the other hand, each individual can sustain his or her appropriate weight by regularly consuming the proper foods in the proper amounts balanced with proper exercise over the course of time.

Food engineering—that is, the alteration of real food to make debased food—is either the main cause or a significant contributing factor in the chronic diseases we discuss in this book. Food engineering is a major focus of Big Food activities. Let us take a closer look.

First, all real food, food as Mother Nature[3] presents it to us—natural food—is health food. Keeping in mind that there are no unmitigated blessings, there is a long list of benefits we derive by controlling nature—controlling *Mother Nature!*—anathema to many, but read on.

When we first emerged as hominins[4] in the Paleolithic Era some two million years ago, we began the process of controlling Mother Nature. We made the first stone knife and spear point, which improved our success in hunting. We continued to increase our control of Mother Nature through the use of fire, animal skin and plant clothing, shelter building, and so on.

The earliest truly major control of nature started with the first agricultural revolution (the Neolithic Revolution) about ten thousand years ago (Richards 2002). Expressed as a percentage of the two million years of hominin existence, the ten thousand-year period from then until now comes to 0.5 percent! Thus, for only 0.5 percent of our existence have we grown the plants we previously foraged, and bred and raised some of the animals we once hunted.

---

3   Mother Nature is a convenient term we use to stand for evolutionary adaptation.

4   The term *hominin*, meaning human ancestor, replaces the earlier term *hominid* to reflect more accurately new genetic findings (Hirst 2010).

Foraging and hunting gave a low return on the invested effort. Bare survival was the best we could get. Even crude, basic agriculture was so efficient by comparison that only some needed to farm, allowing others to build cities; enact laws; and in general, build civilization.

Like all species do when food is plentiful, we increased our population size to the point of starvation for countless people. We were back to basic survival all over again. The control of nature again, this time through the methods of the Green Revolution in the middle of the twentieth century, saved (and is saving) many from hunger, malnutrition, and starvation.

The newly developed agricultural chemicals, plant breeding, and irrigation improvement—Green Revolution methods—allow global food production to keep pace with global population growth (Davies 2003). The father of the revolution, Norman Borlaug, received a Nobel Prize for his efforts.[5]

Some people object to this modern control over Mother Nature, insisting that the food produced under this control is not as nutritionally valuable as food produced organically. However, the argument is flawed; its premise is simply not true. Organic food is as good as, but no better than, any other real food (Magkos, Arvaniti, and Zampelas 2003). Nutritionally, organic food production is similar to the farming methods that prevailed before the Green Revolution. No one will receive a Nobel Prize for suggesting that we go back to the way we were farming in the past—unless the prize foundation decides to open up a new category: marketing.

Let's examine a few basic premises. First, all food is health food until methods of food engineering degrade it. We'll discuss how food is engineered in greater detail later. For now, it's important to know that processing (refining) carbohydrates changes them from real food—health food, if you like—to debased food.

---

5   Food shortages have caused acrimony, fights, and wars. Borlaug, an American agronomist, received the Nobel Peace Prize in 1970 for his contributions to world peace through developing high-yielding crops that prevented starvation for hundreds of millions of people.

It's important to look at the difference between altering food in a minor way and altering it in a major way. When we cook an egg, we alter it from the way Mother Nature gave it to us. We process it. However, cooking alters the egg in a minor way; it coagulates the egg protein. Similarly, cooking meat coagulates its proteins. Coagulated protein is easier to digest. In both examples, we retain important nutrients.

However, when we process sugar cane or sugar beets to make table sugar (sucrose), we alter the cane or the beet in a major way. We keep the sugar and throw away over 90 percent of the cane and the beet! When we process grain to make white flour, we throw away 40 percent of what Mother Nature gave to us. In both cases, we throw away important nutrients (Temple and Burkitt 1993).

Second, sugar, white flour, and engineered fats are the main debased foods. It is nearly impossible to avoid processed carbohydrates and engineered fats today. While scientists might not have the same opinion on all the details, they universally agree on this point: the alteration of real food to make this debased food is either the main cause or a significant contributing factor in the chronic diseases discussed in this book.

Third, the evolutionary perspective plays a role in our food consumption. The introduction of debased foods into our lives is so recent that there is a major disconnect between our original design and our prevailing eating habits. Like all living species, we are wired to blend with the environment of our ancestors. Our genome is that of a lean hunter in a sparse land eating health food only—food as Mother Nature provides it. Debased food appeared only in the last 0.5 percent or less of our existence, and the misfit is serious.

Scientists know that this enormous change in our diet (together with our greatly reduced physical activity) is the main cause for the emergence of the chronic diseases we describe in this book, diseases that were rare in earlier times.

Coincidentally, maintaining good dietary habits over time also benefits mouth health and general health; hence, I have chosen the link between these as the subject of this book. My wish for you? *Oris sana in corpore sano* (a healthy mouth in a healthy body). Now let's explore together how to make that wish a reality.

Bottom Line

1. All real food is health food.
2. Processing (refining) carbohydrates, an important aspect of food engineering, reduces them from real food to debased food.
3. Sugar and white flour (processed carbohydrates) and engineered fats are the main debased foods.
4. From an evolutionary perspective, the introduction of debased foods into our lives is so recent that there is a major inconsistency between our original design and our prevailing eating habits.

Chapter 2.

Carbohydrates: The Misunderstood Energy

Potatoes are fattening and an apple a day keeps the doctor away; the two are common beliefs. In fact, except for their water content, both potatoes and apples are largely carbohydrates, and both are good for us, unless we alter (process or refine) them by peeling them, deep frying them in fat, smothering them in butter, dousing them in caramelized sugar, and so on. As I will show in the last chapter, potatoes, in fact, have a slight dietary edge over apples!

All fruits, vegetables, and grains are mainly carbohydrates and should make up over half of what we eat. They are loaded with vitamins and minerals; they are nutrient dense as opposed to energy dense. *Energy dense* is the scientist's way of saying *fattening*.

Endless myths surround carbohydrates because of their complex chemistry, but the only guide to eating we'll ever need only requires us to know two things about carbohydrates. One, *all* carbs come in just two types—simple and complex. The simple carbs are sugars, and the complex carbs are starches. Except for honey, which is a simple carb, all naturally occurring carbs are a mix of both the simple and the complex types. Two, simple carbs raise blood sugar quickly, and complex carbs raise blood sugar slowly. Quickly is bad; slowly is good. (For more details on carbs and blood sugar, see chapter 12, "The Deadly Quartet: Diabetes.")

Carbohydrates are one of the four macronutrients, along with proteins, lipids, and water. Together with the micronutrients vitamins and minerals, which we need in very small quantities, they comprise all the food we eat. Carbs are stored solar energy, and all living things need energy to function as living things. Reduced to the simple sugar glucose during metabolism, carbohydrates are our primary source of energy. Like fire, technology, and wine, a carbohydrate is a wonderful servant but a terrible master. Used as intended by Mother Nature, carbs make life possible—joys, sorrows, and all. Abused, as they so often are in the developed world, along with engineered fats, they are a major cause of all the chronic diseases of civilization we describe in this book. Dental decay shows up first, and predictably, several decades later, the other ailments—heart disease, diabetes, elevated blood fats, hypertension, excess weight, obesity, constipation, varicose veins, varicocele, hemorrhoids, diverticulitis—follow. Scientists are discovering links between the abuse of food and other diseases as well (Hujoel 2009).

So, how do we abuse carbohydrates? We do so by refining, which is a fancy word for processing, which is a fancy word for degrading.

For the past two hundred years or so, table sugar and white flour have been the primary offenders against Mother Nature. Processing (degrading) sugar beet or sugar cane removes about 90 percent of the beet or cane's nutrients to produce table sugar, and processing wheat removes most of its nutrients to get white flour. To make white flour, Big Food takes most of about *twenty* nutrients out of whole wheat. By requirement of law, the industry then puts *four* of the nutrients back into the flour (Hernot et al. 2008). Because of this reintroduction of the four nutrients, Big Food labels the flour "enriched" (Gunnarsdottir et al. 2009). As unbelievable as this sounds, it's absolutely true.

This processing contributes to dental decay and the other predictable, chronic diseases of civilization in two major ways. First, it removes fiber and micronutrients and, second, it concentrates the sugar. The second is, in part, a result of the first. Removing fiber leads to sugar concentration.

Big Food's record of crimes against sensible eating is long, but the removal of fiber and micronutrients in addition to the concentration of sugar, together with engineered fats, tops the list.

Sugar, an essential nutrient, is not the villain. *Too much* sugar is. The dosage makes the poison. That is true about anything we put in our mouth. The miracle drug, Aspirin, for instance, is the leading cause of poisoning among children. People have taken the vitamins essential for life in toxic doses leading to death. One-millionth of a gram of botulin toxin is fatal. Yet when the quantity is properly adjusted, the same substance treats a large number of muscle problems, wrinkles being the least important. It is not poison when administered in small enough quantities. The dosage makes the poison.

Real food sustains us. When it is converted to engineered food by refining it, it is the leading cause of the chronic diseases that kill us. No one would eat eighteen apples after dinner, but those eighteen apples have the sugar content of one piece of apple pie with a scoop of ice cream, a common enough way of ending dinner. Diffuse, sugar is an important part of the apple that keeps the doctor away. Concentrated, the same sugar is an important part of the apple pie that keeps the doctor busy (Kopp 2003, 2005, 2006) (Sarter, Campbell, and Fuhrman 2008).

Let us look at the diffuse/concentrated phenomenon in a typical hot dog:

- Of a cucumber, 1 percent is sugar; 30 percent of pickle relish is sugar, most of it added.
- Of a tomato, 3 percent is sugar; 25 percent and more of ketchup is sugar, most of it added.
- Of mustard seed, 7 percent is sugar; 40 percent and more of many prepared mustards is sugar, most of it added.
- Of beef, pork, turkey, or chicken, 0 percent is sugar; up to 4 percent of the beef, pork, turkey, or chicken hot dog is sugar, all of it added.

- The micronutrient level of the white flour hot dog bun, even when "enriched," is seriously diminished.

So a nutritionally ideal hot dog could have some sliced cucumber, some sliced tomato, a sprinkling of dry mustard, on top of a small wiener, in a whole wheat bun. That keeps the doctor away.

A commercially ideal hot dog has relish, ketchup, and prepared mustard, on top of a large wiener, in a white bun. That keeps the doctor busy.

Commercially ideal? Yes. Relish has a very long shelf life, as does ketchup, whereas cucumbers and tomatoes spoil quickly. Spoilage is a result of microorganisms "eating" nutritious foods. They are not interested in degraded foods.

White flour buns have a long shelf life. They don't get moldy in a few days. Molds, a life form, are too smart to settle on anything as devoid of nutritional value as a white flour (refined grain) product. They'll go for whole grain products anytime. Should we be taking a lesson from these brainless organisms?

As a survival mechanism, we developed a preference for fats and sugars over millions of years. Through most of our existence, we needed the high energy provided by fats and the quick energy provided by sugars. Our preference for fats and sugars was as essential to continued existence during times of chronic food shortages as it is destructive today, in these times of food abundance.

So the commercially ideal hot dog is made up of ingredients with a long shelf life and with appealing sensory qualities, which add up to eating gratification. Such a hot dog must meet regulatory requirements for safety but not evolutionary standards for health. These are largely absent.

Let us look at other examples of the diffuse/concentrated continuum.

- Of a plum, 10 percent is sugar. Remove much of the water and you get a prune, of which more than 50 percent is sugar.

- Of a grape, 15 percent is sugar. Remove much of the water and you get a raisin, of which 65 percent is sugar.
- Of an apricot, 9 percent is sugar. Remove much of the water and you get a dry apricot, of which over 50 percent is sugar.

Such examples abound.

Prunes, raisins, and dried apricots are not evil, but because of the concentration of their sugars, they are much more likely to do harm if eaten in large quantities, than are plums, grapes, and apricots. The dosage makes the poison.

The history of sugar is fascinating; the increase in people's usage of sugar parallels the development of industrialization. More importantly, people's increased usage of sugar parallels the rise in dental decay, and predictably, a decade or more later, diabetes, elevated blood fats, hypertension, excess weight, and obesity, plus constipation with its consequences (varicose veins, varicocele, hemorrhoids, deep venous thrombosis, and diverticulitis).

An interesting exception to the connection between dental decay and the diseases of civilization is the commonly seen beer belly of serious beer drinkers. The malt sugar in beer is as much a refined carbohydrate as any other sugar and does as much harm when taken excessively. It isn't sweet, so it doesn't taste like sugar and it doesn't interest the mouth bacteria that cause decay.

If we ate sugar in its diffuse, naturally occurring concentration, the doctor, whether a physician or a dentist, would have a lot more time for fishing and golf—a lot more.

In common usage, the term "sugar," the ubiquitous table sugar, applies to sucrose, a simple carb. Anything ending in "-ose" is a sugar, and Mother Nature brings many "-ose" varieties to us in milk, fruits, and vegetables. They never come in high concentration, with the exception of honey which, before the advent of commercial honey production, was rarely a part of the human diet. Sucrose, glucose, fructose, lactose, and maltose (the malt sugar in beer) are a few examples. None are unhealthy in their naturally occurring low concentrations. All are dangerous in their engineered high concentrations, if we eat them as frequently as has become the norm in industrialized societies.

Bottom Line

Unlike in other chapters, there is only one entry here. One single axiom could eliminate most dental decay, and predictably, a decade or more later, all the other diseases of civilization. One law would have such a profound impact on the lives of all people who have adopted a Western diet that we should elevate it to a commandment: *Thou shalt not refine carbohydrates.*

In the westernized world of today, that would be difficult. However, in our own lives, we can significantly reduce our intake of these harmful refined carbohydrates by simply changing a few habits. We can eliminate sugar from our coffee or tea (Malik et al. 2006); stop consuming soft drinks, sugared juices, "energy" drinks, and foods with added sugars (any with added ingredients ending in "-ose") and choosing whole grains instead of "enriched" breads. Each of these is doable, and each will be satisfying once we get over old habits.

Chapter 3.

Proteins: Life's Blueprint

Proteins are another of the four macronutrient categories indispensable to good nutrition. They have had an important role in most biologic functions, structures, and energy sources from the very beginning of life. Not only are proteins part of the makeup of hormones, hormone receptors, RNA, DNA, enzymes, neurotransmitters, and more, they play a vital role in the functionality of each of these (Haimel, Pröll and Rebhan 2009).

In their structural role, proteins are a major constituent of bone, muscle, blood, even teeth (Sire et al. 2007), as well as other tissues and tissue fluids. As an energy source, the body uses proteins only if it cannot get enough calories from the two other sources at its disposal, namely carbohydrates and fats. Protein molecules tend to be bigger than carbohydrate molecules, so the body needs more time to digest them. Consequently, they are a longer-lasting energy source than carbohydrates, which probably explains why low-carb weight loss diets are effective, albeit temporarily.

Since proteins make up some aspect of all living things, and since everything we eat was or still is living (fresh fruit and vegetables are alive), proteins are not hard to come by whatever we eat. However, the millions and millions of proteins that exist are all made of only twenty building blocks called amino acids, and our bodies can make only about half of these from raw materials in our diet. The other half, called essential amino acids, must come from the food we eat. Animal source proteins (all meat, milk, and eggs) are complete proteins because they contain all twenty amino acids. Fruits and vegetables have negligible amounts of protein, but wheat, corn, rice, and beans are good plant sources of proteins. However, except for soybeans and soy products, plant proteins are incomplete. They are missing some of the essential amino acids. Nonetheless, the right juggling can get around that easily.

Strict vegetarians are good at eating the right combinations of foods to ensure they get complete proteins without animal proteins (Craig and Mangels 2009). Looking into the diets of hundreds of patients convinced me that typical vegetarians are exceptionally nutritionally aware, however uninteresting their diets appear to people like me.

The balanced diet[6]* provides daily protein needs effortlessly, so we hardly need to think about proteins. Further, it is almost impossible to get too much protein, so we can go on to other issues.

An interesting recent discovery, confirmed after extensive studies, is that a family of proteins found in milk (casein phosphopeptides, for the curious) prevents dental decay and, in fact, reverses it in early cases (Ferrazzano et al. 2008). Is it a choice between brushing or a piece of cheese? Is cheddar better (Barbour et al. 2008)? Actually, it is not a choice; we need to eat beneficial foods *and* brush after meals in order to clean our teeth and gums. Together with flossing, regular dental checkups and cleanings combined with eating as this book recommends, we can maintain general and dental health, have a bright smile and fresh breath, and minimize health expenses.

Bottom Line

1. A balanced diet will effortlessly provide all the proteins we need.

---

6 • A balanced diet has the appropriate amount and mix of macronutrients and micronutrients to meet an individual's ongoing nutritional needs.

2. With informed awareness of which foods provide complementary amino acid sources, a vegetarian diet can also provide all of the essential amino acids.

3. Soybeans and soybean products are the only common plant sources containing all twenty amino acids. They are nutritionally outstanding.

4. Protein supplements do a lot more good for the seller than for the buyer. Protein shortages in the developed world simply don't exist.

5. In addition to being excellent nutritionally, milk products can protect against tooth decay and even reverse decay in its early stages.

Chapter 4.

Fats: Love Them, You Can't Leave Them

Surveys repeatedly reveal a great deal of confusion about fats and fat labeling (Eckel et al. 2009). Not only are consumers unsure what fats are and what labeling means, they don't trust Big Food for reliable information—and for good reasons. Industry interests are frequently not aligned with consumer interests; marketers confuse consumers with clever advertising and wording that promotes their products in misleading ways. Engineered food—that is, food that our grandparents would not recognize—is engineered in the interest of the food industry.

Let us demystify fats. Fats and oils are collectively called lipids. They are one of the four macronutrient groups (the others being carbohydrates, proteins, and water) and are indispensable for good health (Ascherio and Willett 1997). Lipids are vital for fetal development; children's growth; absorption of vitamins A, D, E, and K; and maintenance of skin health, and they play a role in regulating many other metabolic functions. They also insulate the body and support and pad organs.

Weight control and heart health are the two concerns most people have with dietary fat, and rightly so (Ascherio et al. 1996).

However, the notion that fat will make us fat is a misconception, mathematically speaking. As we will discuss in chapter 10, "The Deadly Quartet: Excess Weight and Obesity," the body understands grade school arithmetic only. Food of any kind will make us fat if we eat more than we need. The source of calories is irrelevant.

Having said that, we do need to be aware of the fact that, at 9 calories per gram, *all* fats, and that includes oils, have more than *twice* the number of calories of an equal measure of proteins or carbohydrates, which have 4 calories each. Alcohol, not a nutrient, is the other source of dietary calories and has 7 calories per gram. Fats are the most concentrated source of energy in the diet, whether they are:

1) saturated
2) trans fats
3) mono*un*saturated
4) poly*un*saturated
5) omega-3 fatty acids
6) omega-6 fatty acids
7) any other lipids

Making a distinction between these types of lipids is vital if you are a scientist studying fats on a molecular level. For the rest of us, the distinction is unimportant as far as weight control is concerned.

What we do need to recognize when looking at the role of fats in weight control is that we are wired to love fats. During the first 99.5 percent of humanity's existence most of us constantly faced food shortages. For reasons of survival, we had to favor the most energy-dense (fattening) aspects of whatever food we came across. Fats are at the top of the list.

When it comes to heart health, unlike weight control concerns, the distinction between the fat groups is critical. In that respect, not all fats are created equal. There are good fats and bad fats, and all are a mix of many different fatty acids. How these fatty acids are linked together determines whether the fats are unsaturated or saturated.

I italicized the *un* in the list of lipid types to help us identify the good ones. We need to avoid or minimize items 1) and 2)—trans fats and saturated fats. The others are good fats and are important for good health. They should add up to about one-third of our daily calories, with most coming from oils found in nuts, fish, and vegetable oils—olive, corn, canola, safflower, soybean, and sunflower.

Avoiding saturated fats altogether is neither necessary nor possible because most fats are a mix of several of the above groups. All occur in nature. However, most trans fats on our grocery shelves are engineered. They can be made cheaply, stored cheaply, handled cheaply, transported cheaply, and have a long shelf life—all the qualities that the food industry looks for. On the subject of fats, respected diet experts worldwide universally agree that minimizing our intake of saturated fats and avoiding trans fats is all we need to do for maximal health (Mensink and Katan 1990) (Motoyama et al. 2009).

A Word about Cholesterol

Cholesterol is actually an alcohol. (All compounds ending in "ol" belong to the alcohol family.) But cholesterol is a fatlike substance, so we include it in the chapter on fats. Cholesterol plays an important role in many physiological functions and structures, and the body manufactures most of it. If we never got any from our diet, cholesterol would still be present in our bodies to work at its many normal jobs.

While some cholesterol in the bloodstream is vital, more definitely isn't better. In fact, a surplus can lead to a buildup in blood vessel walls, reduce blood flow to arteries, and lead to a heart attack or stroke (Ascherio et al. 1996). Heart disease is the leading cause of death in the Western world.

Dietary cholesterol is found only in animal foods, such as egg yolks, butter, organ meats, beef, chicken, and shellfish. Vegetable oils are cholesterol free.

Your Mouth, Your Health Connection

In addition to weight control and heart health concerns, high-fat diets tend to be low in the complex carbohydrates so necessary for mouth health and general health. As an example, while Canadians enjoy among the longest life expectancy in the world, the Inuit, a subset of the Canadian population, have the lifespan of the developing world—more than twelve years shorter than other Canadians (Government of Canada 2008). The Inuit diet is exceptionally low in complex carbohydrates. While, at this time, there are no high-quality studies of Inuit life expectancy—that is, studies that control for smoking, alcoholism, and other important variables— to confirm a correlation between diet and lifespan, it is reasonable to hypothesize that the lack of complex carbohydrates could be part of the explanation.

Bottom Line

1. Diets high in any fats are energy dense and create weight-control challenges.
2. Diets high in saturated fats and trans fats increase the risk of heart disease.
3. The good fats (fats other than saturated or trans fats) keep our hearts healthy.
4. Much of the increased risk of high-fat diets is the end result of associated decreased intake of unrefined carbohydrates and their fiber content.
5. The benefits of reducing dietary saturated fats and trans fats are likely to be small, unless accompanied by an increased consumption of unrefined carbohydrates.
6. About a third of our calories should come from healthy fats.
7. Fats inhibit stomach emptying more than other macronutrients. They stave off hunger longer.
8. For more on fats, see the Canadian and the USA Web sites www.hc-sc.gc.ca/fn-an/index-eng.php and www.mypyramid.gov. Both sites provide reliable, science-based information that is free of commercial bias.

Chapter 5.

Water: Need Turned to Marketing Triumph

You wouldn't think so to look at us, but we are mostly made of water. About 60 percent of our total body weight is water (plus or minus 15 percent, depending on the amount of body fat a person has—fatty tissues are less than 10 percent water, so more fat equals less water making up our total body weight). Even bone is nearly 25 percent water.

Life originated in water. The earliest single-celled organisms were bathed in water and absorbed dissolved nutrients from ancient oceans, the "primordial soup."[7] The metabolic wastes from those organisms then went back into the soup. Our cells today are bathed in water and absorb very similar dissolved nutrients from the bloodstream and cerebrospinal fluid, the evolved equivalent of the primordial soup. The wastes from this process go back into those fluids to be removed.

All life needs an ongoing supply of water. For most of our evolutionary history, humans drank nothing but water after being weaned. Clean, fresh drinking water continues to be an important

---

7   In 1924, Alexander Oparin, a Russian biochemist, proposed the theory
     that life on earth developed through slow evolution of carbon-based
     molecules in a primordial soup (Fry 2006).

bodily requirement to support life. However, most of us today drink less water than we should, opting instead for high-calorie and high-sugar soft drinks, energy drinks, juices, and the like. This is largely responsible for the alarming increase in weight gain and outright obesity in developed nations (Gyntelberg 2009) (Bray 2008) (Wolf, Bray, and Popkin 2008). To be perfectly clear, *nothing* beats pure, clean water for its health benefits to our bodies. Water has no calories and costs next to nothing. Bottled water is a marketing ploy. In developed nations, it is not necessary to drink bottled water, except during disasters or emergencies or if untested well water is the only other option. For the majority of us living in towns and cities today, the treated water that comes from our taps is as safe and healthy as expensive and environmentally unfriendly bottled water (Doria 2006) (Gualberto and Heller 2006). I'll discuss this further, later.

Water is an essential macronutrient, along with carbohydrates, proteins, and fats. Just as we require an adequate supply of food containing appropriate amounts of carbs, proteins, and fats, we also need adequate hydration at all times to remain alive and healthy.

The Benefits of Water

1. Water delivers nutrients to the cells of our bodies and takes away the wastes of metabolism.
2. Water helps maintain normal blood pressure.
3. Water helps regulate body temperature.
4. Water is an important component of synovial fluid, which lubricates and cushions joints.
5. Water is contained in the fluids that protect our organs.
6. Water is a key element of saliva, which initiates the digestion of starches, keeps the soft tissues of the mouth healthy, and helps control the bacteria that cause cavities.

How to Stay Hydrated

The best replacement for water lost during metabolism is water—not soft drinks, beer, coffee, or wine. Having said that, studies show that *modest* alcohol and coffee consumption offers some health benefits. Modest is the key word here (Knoops 2004). Coffee and alcoholic beverages are diuretics, meaning they cause increased urination. We lose more water than we take in by drinking these. Tea is the exception—unless it has sugar in it, tea is a good way to replace lost water.

Fruits and vegetables contain a large percentage of water. Eating fruits and vegetables as snacks and at mealtimes is a good way to stay hydrated. Soups and juices also contribute to our water needs. However, we need to keep in mind that most packaged soups and juices are engineered products. They usually have large amounts of sodium as well as sugar. Either make soups and juices yourself or read labels carefully.

How Much is Enough

Both Canadian and U.S. government agencies recommend daily water intake based on age and gender. However, these are difficult to monitor due to variations in ambient temperatures, varying levels of activity among individuals, and varying sources of water other than water itself. Urine color and thirst are more reliable indicators that you are sufficiently hydrated.

Urine Color and Odor – Urine that is odorless and colorless or light yellow is a good indicator of adequate hydration.

Thirst – Thirst indicates that we are already a bit dehydrated. As we get older, thirst is an increasingly poor indicator of our need for water (Kenney and Chiu 2001). We should rehydrate on an ongoing basis and more so during hot weather or periods of exertion. We should keep a glass of water by our bedside to rehydrate during the night.

Water and Dental Issues

Every dentist regularly sees patients with state-of-the-art, sophisticated, and expensive crown and bridgework (caps, veneers, fixed bridges) that are failing, sometimes after more than two decades of function, because of rampant, sudden onset of tooth root decay. Actually, the bridgework doesn't fail—its support does!

> Example 1. A charming lady in her eighties, whose bridgework required us to cap *every* tooth some twenty-five years earlier, comes in for her regular checkup. A quick screening examination shows several unexpected areas of decay under some of the crowns so we decide to do a full mouth survey—we X-ray *all* the teeth. The initial look at the X-rays as they come out of the developer confirms what we dreaded. The presence of recurrent decay is everywhere. Her bridgework is doomed.

> Example 2. An elderly man, a patient in our office for decades, phones to ask for an urgent appointment to have us re-cement his upper front, six-tooth bridge. It came off as he bit into a sandwich. We know from bitter experience that this is not a case of cement failure. Rather, the teeth supporting the bridge broke off—failed physically—because of recurrent decay. The bridge has no future.

> Example 3. We compliment a patient on the fact that, at age fifty, he has no fillings and no cavities. Many baby boomers fit this description, thanks to improved dental hygiene. However, two years later, this patient develops a life-threatening condition needing daily medication that dries up normal salivary flow. Three years after that, he loses *all* his teeth because of untreatable, advanced, generalized rampant decay.

What common thread do these examples share? Why, after an enduring, problem-free period of health, do the roots of these teeth decay?

Xerostomia is the answer. Not an everyday word, *xerostomia* simply means dry mouth. To some extent, it affects one out of four people and is a common feature of normal aging. Additionally, medication causes a lot of xerostomia, with over four hundred common prescription drugs listing dry mouth as a side effect. Some diseases contribute as well. Researchers have explored diabetes, lupus, kidney disease, stress, anxiety, depression, nutritional deficiencies, and immune system problems in depth and published hundreds of scholarly papers on the role of these diseases in xerostomia (Thelin et al. 2008). Trauma resulting in nerve damage to the head and neck is another common cause of dry mouth, as is radiation treatment in the area of the salivary glands.

In addition to diminishing the flavor of foods, dry mouth is frequently the primary cause of the dental problems described above. The type of decay xerostomia causes under crowns and bridges can be very difficult to treat. Implants take more effort to maintain and can also fail.

To Control Dry Mouth

- Sip water frequently.
- Avoid sugary foods and drinks (be aware that anything on an ingredient label that ends in "-ose" is a sugar—sucrose, fructose, and so forth).
- Chew sugar-free gum.
- Use lip moisturizers.
- Humidify the air at home.
- Use toothpaste that contains fluoride.
- Brush at least four times a day (after each meal and before bedtime).
- Apply prescription-strength fluoride gel at bedtime, as prescribed, or chew fluoride lozenges as prescribed.
- If your case is extreme, your dentist or physician can prescribe a salivary stimulant drug.

Water and Diet

Because water, one of the four essential macronutrients, has no calories, filling up on water does not satisfy hunger. We are wired that way for survival. If filling up on water satisfied hunger, we'd miss out on the calories essential for survival, the calories we get from eating the other three essential macronutrients.

Similarly, filling up on calorie-loaded soft drinks does not satisfy hunger. We don't eat any less at the next meal. If we take in a 250-calorie snack, we will eat that much less at our next meal without even thinking about it. That is not so if the calories come from soft drinks. We will consume these calories in addition to, not instead of, the food calories we consume during the next meal. When your body has more calories than it needs to perform the activities you're requiring of it, you have a positive energy balance (extra calories). The opposite (too few calories) creates a negative energy balance.

It is a mathematical certainty that, over time, even a small positive energy balance will result in weight gain. See "The Deadly Quartet" chapters for details.

Bottled Water

Untreated drinking water has caused an untold number of epidemics and poisonings throughout history and still does so. Our fear of poisoning by drinking water is primordial and goes back to our earliest origins. However, today, most industrialized nations can be proud of the safety of their drinking water. A search of government health sites in North America[8] demonstrates that rigorous standards are in place to ensure municipal water safety. Safe public drinking water is a major reason for the near doubling of life expectancy during the twentieth century. The safe and secure provision of water to millions of people living in our towns and cities is one of the major public health triumphs of the last century (Morse 2007).

---

8   U.S. Food and Drug Administration, located at http://www.fda.gov/, and Health Canada, located at http://www.hc-sc.gc.ca.

On the other hand, bottled water is one of the major *marketing* triumphs of the last century. Much of bottled water is just packaged tap water. It is neither safer nor better for us. In this glaring example of the victory of marketing over science, bottled water marketers lead many consumers to believe that bottled water is safer than the water coming out of their taps.

The economics of buying bottled water are astonishing. First, the consumer pays for the installation, maintenance, and operation of municipal water in the community. Then the bottlers take the water from that sophisticated, paid-for supply; add their packaging, transportation, storage, and (the biggest of all) marketing costs; and sell it back to that same consumer at a grossly inflated markup of several thousand times the original cost. At well over $1.50 per 500-mL bottle, this water costs over $3.00 per liter—much more expensive than the gas we put in our vehicles!

We need to think before we drink.

If You Are on a Well

Governments ensure safe and secure public water supply for the 90 percent of us who have access to it. If you are among the 10 percent of North Americans who get water from wells, governments will test it for you any time you send in a sample. Since well water is affected by runoff, which changes with spills, pesticides, and other occasional influences, its safety is your responsibility.

If you get your water from a well, using bottled water for drinking makes sense.

Bottom Line

1. If you drink up to six cups of coffee a day, plus two glasses of wine or two pints of beer, you will derive some proven, although minor, health benefits (Knoops 2004).
2. If you drink soda pop and energy drinks in moderation, you will develop some proven, although minor health

damage. If you drink a lot you'll pay a high price. Damage to health is directly proportional to intake.

3. Fruit juices are refined products from which the roughage has been removed. Drinking them in moderation won't hurt if they have no sugar or preservatives added, but eating the fruit from which they are derived is better. Most juices have no pectin, the fruit equivalent of fiber.

4. We were designed to satisfy our thirst with water and not with soda pop, energy drinks, juices, coffee, or alcoholic beverages. Straying from our original design is harmful in direct proportion to the degree to which we stray.

Chapter 6.

Vitamins and Minerals: Need Turned to Hoax

Vitamins and minerals are micronutrients, and together with water and the macronutrients (carbohydrates, proteins, and fats) are essential to good eating. We couldn't live without them. But like so much in life, the right balance is crucial.

Since we've given vitamin C a lot of attention in the last few decades, let's start with it.

Hippocrates was the first to describe a disease called scurvy in 400 BC. Resulting from a deficiency in vitamin C, scurvy was a debilitating disease that plagued many during long, hard winters and sailors during lengthy sea voyages. Hippocrates's description might well have been the first connection between the lack of a nutrient and its corresponding deficiency disease.

In the middle of the nineteenth century, during an extended sea voyage, James Lind, a British Royal Navy surgeon, gave oranges and lemons to a group of sailors, along with their usual rations, while another group did not get the fruit. The results conclusively showed that citrus fruits prevented scurvy, and Lind published his findings. This was the first published, controlled experiment in science that compared the effect of one variable on a selected group of subjects to a similar group that was missing that variable (Bartholomew 2002).

As a result, the British admiralty began supplying limes or their juice as a part of sailors' rations for sea voyages. When these sailors came to the New World, Americans and Canadians observed this practice of sucking on limes and soon applied the slang nickname "limey" to the British.

But while the connection between food and health was long established, it was Linus Pauling's 1970 book, *Vitamin C and the Common Cold*, that really began the craze that sees people using vitamin supplements for improved health.[9] Few books have stirred so much hope for so many. Nearly forty years after it first appeared in print, Pauling's controversial book continues to spawn imitators and wannabes of all sorts. However, few books have annoyed nutrition scientists as much. The majority disagree with Pauling, who claimed that taking 1,000 milligrams of vitamin C daily would reduce the incidence of the common cold by 45 percent. That claim is testable, but Pauling never tested it rigorously. Others did. Numerous studies have looked for the benefits of large vitamin C doses and found none. One meta-analysis,[10] which reported on thirty trials looking at 11,350 participants, examined the relative risk of developing a cold while taking preventive doses of vitamin C. The analysis concluded "Routine mega-dose prophylaxis is not rationally justified" (Douglas 2007). Another study, in fact, showed that high doses of vitamin C reduce the effectiveness the most commonly used antineoplastic drugs in the treatment of cancer patients (Heaney et al. 2008).

In the absence of any clear, scientific proof that vitamin C or other micronutrient supplementation has a therapeutic or preventative impact on our health, we should follow the lead of our healthy hunter–gatherer ancestors, who got all of their vitamins

---

9   Pauling's credentials as a scientist are impeccable. An influential writer, teacher, and scientist, he twice won the Nobel Prize (for chemistry in 1954 and for peace in 1962) and nearly won the race against Crick and Watson to describe the DNA molecule, which would have given him a third. He has few equals in twentieth-century science, and this reputation made the book an instant best seller.

10   A review of all high-quality science papers on one topic is referred to as a meta-analysis. In science circles, this is considered to be the mother of all scientific reviews.

and minerals, including vitamin C, from the foods they ate. Real food has many micronutrients that supplements do not, certainly including some that have yet to be discovered.

Physician-prescribed, patient-specific supplements are another matter. Pregnant women benefit from daily supplementation with a multivitamin that contains folic acid in the patient-specific dose recommended by their physicians (Blencowe et al. 2010). Elderly people should take 700–800 mg of calcium and 400–800 IU of vitamin D per day (Gennari 2001). Research has not effectively demonstrated consumer health benefits of vitamin and mineral supplements, apart from these two exceptions (Johnson and Landry 1998).

Excessive use of supplements, in fact, can have serious, even fatal, results. Arctic explorers have died from eating polar bear liver, which has toxic levels of vitamin A. Few of us will ever eat polar bear liver, but it is possible to overdose on vitamin A supplements available at the corner drug store. In 2007, *The Journal of the American Medical Association* reported a review of *all* high-quality studies of vitamin A supplementation published to date, a meta-analysis, and concluded that treatment with beta carotene, vitamin A, and vitamin E may *increase* mortality (Bjelakovic et al. 2008). The increase is slight, but nonetheless, it is an increase.

These are facts. Yet half the population takes nonprescription supplements. This is the triumph of marketing over science. The benefits to supplement sellers are clear. They serve a market of innocents, hopefuls, charlatans, quacks, and cultists. The objective of marketing is to persuade; the objective of science is to discover truth. Medical literature urges clinicians to emphasize the importance of a proper diet to their younger patients and not to encourage supplement use (Briefel et al. 2006).

The advantages of protein supplements are even more spurious. Eating proteins in the form of supplements amounts to displacing important nutrients present in food from Mother Nature's cupboard with engineered foods. It benefits the vendor alone.

The best advice: Comply with recommendations specifically made for you by physicians and dietitians and beware those who recommend multivitamin and multimineral supplements who also sell these products. Recognize the inherent conflict of interest in the latter situation.

Scientists who study nutrition know that eating the way Mother Nature designed us to eat—that is, eating the way hunters and gatherers ate—provides all the natural carbohydrates, proteins, fats, vitamins, minerals, and water that we need.

As part of my research for *Your Mouth, Your Health*, I examined food guides and pyramids of many advanced nations. Each of these guides—all science-based—supports the position that foods (in a balanced diet) *without supplementation* will provide us with all our nutrient needs, as do science-based vegetarian and vegan food pyramids.

A Word about Sodium[11]

Sodium is a micronutrient—one of hundreds. So why single out sodium instead of any of the others? Like many other micronutrients, sodium was an important part of the primordial cell's ocean environment. It remains important in the environment of all living cells today, be they a complete organism in and of themselves or a part of a complex, multicellular organism. Abundant in the oceans in the form of sodium chloride, sodium is rare inland. So, for survival reasons, we love sodium just as much as we love fats and sugars, the other two essential and rare basic nutrients. All three were critical and hard to come by during most of our existence.[12]

---

11 Most of the sodium in our food comes in the form of table salt, and the two words are commonly used interchangeably. To chemists, table salt is sodium chloride. There are other sources of sodium, such as sodium bicarbonate (baking soda), monosodium glutamate (MSG), and so on. For our purposes, we can think of sodium as being table salt.

12 Carnivores meet their sodium needs from the tissues and tissue fluids of their prey. Herbivores like deer, moose, elephants, woodchucks, porcupines, mountain goats, domestic sheep, cattle, and a long list of other animals seek out salty mineral deposits exposed by harsh weather conditions.

That is why the combination of salt, fat, and sugar is irresistible. The ancient Romans understood the mouth-watering power of this titillating trio and frequently used it in their cooking. Science today understands the anatomic, hormonal, neurologic, psychological, and social forces involved (Frassetto et al. 2001) (Kurlansky 2002). Big Food understands how to adapt the forces behind the titillating trio into the irresistible, terrible trio of engineered foods that we can't stop eating. Big Food's twist on the trio is one of the major causes of the epidemic of excess weight and obesity today (Kessler 2009). Big Food puts the terrible trio into nearly everything they make.

This irresistible, terrible trio would be fully neutralized if we observed the bottom line in chapter 2: *Thou shalt not refine carbohydrates.*

Facts about Fluoride

You don't expect to read a chapter on supplements by a dentist without hearing about fluoride, do you?

The bottom line on this issue, not a contentious one among scientists, is that optimal levels of fluoride help build and maintain strong and healthy hard tissues, namely tooth enamel and dentin and every bone and every cartilage surface in our bodies (Brown 1965). Looking at hard numbers, one comprehensive study concluded that "water fluoridation offers significant cost savings" (Griffin et al. 2001). The dollar savings in reducing bone and joint disease are incalculable. The quality of life improvement cannot be measured in dollars.

The Centers for Disease Control and Prevention (CDC) lists fluoridation of municipal water as one of the great public health triumphs of the twentieth century (Centers for Disease Control and Prevention 1999). That puts it in the same league with vaccination; measures improving motor vehicle safety; safer workplaces; control of infectious diseases; safer and healthier foods; healthier mothers and babies; the decline in deaths from coronary heart disease and stroke; family planning; and recognition of tobacco use as a health hazard.

All dental and public health organizations worldwide support fluoridation of public water supplies and consider it a safe and effective measure. Why, then, is fluoridation of municipal water so controversial among the well informed and misinformed? Governmental bodies add fluoride to public water supplies, thus imposing fluoride on everyone. Therefore fluoridation becomes another example of an age-old conflict—individual rights versus the common good.

There are many ways to benefit from optimal fluoride levels but the most common, reliable source is public water supply. Your dentist will recommend optimal fluoride supplements and topical dental applications adjusted for the fluoride levels in your community water and for your specific needs if you are not among the 70 percent of the population that enjoys the health benefits of fluoridation.

Bottom Line

1. Vitamins and minerals are nutrients, and in the vast majority of cases, eating a variety of foods rich in vitamins and minerals is preferable to self-prescribing large doses of vitamins and minerals in the form of supplements.

2. Eat as recommended by the science-based food guides provided by the United States and Canada[13]. Such a diet will provide all the vitamins and minerals you need.(I've included additional food guide information in chapter 15.)

3. Unless a qualified professional recommends supplementation to what you eat, unless you are pregnant or nursing, and unless you are elderly, don't waste your money on supplements.

4. Look for the irresistible, terrible trio (salt, fat, and sugar) that Big Food includes in nearly all engineered food it markets aggressively. In moderation, the terrible trio is

13 Find the United States' food guides at http://www.mypyramid.gov/ and Canada's at http://www.hc-sc.gc.ca/fn-an/food-guide-aliment/ index-eng.php.

harmless, but in excess, the trio can cause or contribute to some very serious health issues. Part of what makes the combination so deadly is its addictiveness: moderation is easier said than done.

5. Find out from your municipality whether your water is fluoridated. If you live among the 30 percent of the population where community water isn't fluoridated, ask your dentist for fluoride supplements for your very young children. If your grandchildren or other young children you know live in one of these areas encourage their parents to talk to their dentist. Systemic fluoride is of little dental value after teeth have finished forming.

Chapter 7.

Origins: Food for Thought

If one hour represents our existence as *Homo sapiens*, then the Industrial Revolution began less than half a second ago.

How much did a one hundred-year-old tree grow in the last four days? The ratio is the same.[14] Now, the growth of the one hundred-year-old tree during those four days is as imperceptible as is the change in its environment. The changes in our bodies during the last half second of the hour of our existence is similarly imperceptible; the changes that took place in our environment during the same half a second were more than colossal—they were catastrophic.

Like all dentists, in my daily practice, I constantly see the aftermath of the mismatch from a dental perspective. Dentists have seen it since dentistry began (Starling and Stock 2007). In

---

14 For the mathematically inquisitive, scientists generally agree that *Homo sapiens* arose as a distinct species about two million years ago and that the Industrial Revolution began about two hundred years ago. Expressed as a percentage of our total existence, the period from the Industrial Revolution to current times represents 0.01 percent. Each hour contains 3,600 seconds, and 0.01 percent of 3,600 equals .36 of a second. Rounded, we can call it half a second.

As to the growth of the tree, one hundred years contains 36,500 days, and 0.01 percent of that equals 3.65 days. Rounded, we can say it comes to four days.

Your Mouth, Your Health, I hope to show how we can, nonetheless, achieve harmony.

Just like all species, we are designed, built, and wired to fit into the environment of our ancestors (Eaton, Konner and Shostak 1988). Our nutritional and activity requirements date from before the Stone Age (Eaton and Eaton 2003). Our biology is ancient and genetically determined to allow us to achieve reproductive success by blending into the environment our ancestors knew millions of years ago (Richards 2002). The colossal changes in that environment began about ten thousand years ago when our ancestors learned to cultivate the soil to produce crops and breed animals as a food source, and intensified exponentially with the Industrial Revolution about two hundred years ago. The result is that our industrialized Western lifestyle is profoundly discordant with our genetic makeup. It is at odds with our design because it is a major and a very recent development from an evolutionary perspective; there is no hope that we could adjust in such a short timeframe.

The misfit between our ancient design, build, and wiring and modern-day, Westernized nutritional and activity habits has resulted in an alarming rise in the diseases of civilization (Eaton 2006). The biologic functions of the macro- and micronutrient food groups, which we touched on in preceding chapters, have not changed one iota since the beginning of time. However, the composition and packaging of macronutrients (carbohydrates, proteins, fats, and water) has undergone incredible, profit-motivated changes as Big Food has moved them from natural to engineered forms.

Micronutrient composition, on the other hand, is the same as ever because the smallest change would make micronutrients useless. Regulatory agencies would not allow Big Food to engineer or alter these two food groups (vitamins and minerals).

To achieve profit-motivated objectives with micronutrients, Big Food has resorted to attractive but meaningless packaging and fear mongering. They market micronutrients as "supplements" and instill in consumers the fear that, without supplementation, they will miss out on something that is hugely beneficial.

The fact is that unless they are recommended by a qualified professional, the best that can be said about "supplements" is that they are mostly harmless to the consumer and profitable for the vendor. (See chapter 6, "Vitamins and Minerals: Need Turned to Hoax.")

The impact of these massive changes in our environment during that last half a second ranges from the strongly positive to the strongly negative—a double-edged sword.

On the positive side (to name just a few of the many changes), this last half a second has seen:

- The doubling of lifespan compared to the first fifty-nine and a half minutes
- Worldwide effective and instant communication with tremendously enhanced access to information for and education of the masses
- The end of distance through the advent of transportation vehicles unthinkable before this time

On the negative side (again, to name just a few of the changes), this time period has given rise to:

- Crowd behavior in markets and related economic traumas
- Road rage
- Turf protection, most egregiously expressed as war

The negative behaviors we've exhibited in the last half a second are flagrantly, insidiously destructive—the eating patterns which result in diet-related health problems are no less so than the aggression and violence.

Two factors in the design/use misfit combine to add up to the alarming incidence and prevalence[15] of the many chronic diseases of civilization.

---

15 In biostatistics, *incidence* refers to newly diagnosed cases of a disease while *prevalence* refers to the number of people who have it. So, diabetes has a low yearly incidence but a high prevalence, whereas a flu epidemic can have a high yearly incidence but a low prevalence.

1. During all but that last half second of our existence as a species, we lived under conditions of food scarcity and privation. There was a substantial survival advantage to the "see food" diet. See food, eat food.

2. Even though our diets always varied according to geography and climate, there was one major universal quality to them all – they were not engineered and degraded by processing or refining.

Through natural selection, evolution is a constant interaction between an organism's genome (characteristics that are passed on from parent to offspring) and its environment. It is important for us to view both the availability and the quality of today's food as important components of that environment. How an individual organism's genome fits its environment determines its survival prospects and reproductive success.

Most often, environments change slowly, allowing many, but not all, living organisms to adapt to the changes. When environments change permanently, unless previously fit individuals adapt in parallel with that change, they become unfit. Genome–environment harmony becomes genome–environment discord. Organisms that don't adapt become extinct. [16]

Continuous genome–environment dissonance on an individual basis most certainly leads to premature extinction of that individual. However, the good news is that, as individuals, we have total control over how we personally mesh our diets and activities to produce harmony with our environment, when all around us we see the appalling results of a mismatch. And more good news is that it is never too late to start.

Bottom Line

1. The misfit between the way we are designed and the way we live is serious.

---

16 As a matter of interest, many more plant and animal species are extinct than are in existence and *Homo sapiens* had nothing to do with a very large percentage of that extinction.

2. Collectively for us in the Western world, health prospects are declining.
3. Individually, however, we are in charge.
4. We are free to embrace a healthy lifestyle. We simply need to:
5. Know and follow "The Only Guide to Eating You'll Ever Need."

PART II

AVOIDABLE CHRONIC DISEASES

Chapter 8.

Dental Decay: The Preventable Scourge

Endless debate surrounds Mona Lisa's smile. Is it the result of Leonardo da Vinci's erotic fixation with his mother's smile or a self-portrait of the artist in drag? Is it a product of sleep deprivation because of the recent arrival of Mona Lisa's second son or is it something else entirely?

Dental historians don't speculate along these lines at all. They know that, like most of her contemporaries, Mona Lisa did not have much to smile with. The next time you are in front of a magazine rack displaying dozens of "eye candy" publications featuring faces of beautiful people, note that more than half of them display teeth, each one perfect. Conversely, the next time you are in an art gallery or looking through an illustrated fine art book featuring faces of historically important people, note that *none* display teeth, perfect or otherwise.

Why is this so? Before modern dentistry most people's teeth, if present, were ugly because of poor hygiene and poor nutrition, resulting in decay and gum disease. Thanks to modern dentistry, we now see the bright, attractive smile everywhere. It is a key factor in personal success.

The branch of modern dentistry most responsible for the Hollywood smile is called *restorative* dentistry within the profession. What are we restoring? We are bringing teeth back to an earlier and better condition from which they strayed, most often as a result of decay. Other reasons for the need for restorative dentistry are trauma, congenital abnormalities, and iatrogenic factors,[17] but decay and its consequences top the list.

The dental decay giving rise to the need for restorative dentistry is, itself, a product of modern times.

As I noted in the chapter on carbohydrates (chapter 2), what Big Food calls refining I call degrading—the industry strips these foods of their fiber and nutrient content. Dental decay results when bacteria interact with one of these "refined" carbohydrates, mainly sugars. We supply the sugars to the bacteria by eating the sugars. White flour and white rice are the other degraded carbohydrates that play a major role in the chronic diseases of civilization we deal with in his book. Before the advent of agriculture, there were no degraded carbohydrates.

Tooth decay results from a four-step chain reaction:

Step 1. The consumption of sugar, a degraded carbohydrate, starts the sequence of events, especially if the sugar sticks to teeth.

Step 2. The metabolic action of bacteria on this sugar produces an acid.

Step 3. The acid begins to dissolve the structure of tooth enamel. At this point, the process is still reversible.

Step 4. The acid dissolution continues on into the dentin of the tooth and may penetrate the nerve. From here on, the matter gets more serious: nerve death and, before modern dentistry, often the death of the owner of the tooth completes the process.

---

17 *Iatrogenic* is derived from the Greek word *iatros* meaning "healer" and stands for adverse conditions caused inadvertently by professional treatment. A few examples of iatrogenic symptoms are an allergic response caused by medication; lethargy, vomiting, and hair loss caused by cancer treatment; stomach bleeding caused by anti-inflammatory medication; liver damage caused by pain pills; and staining of teeth caused by tetracycline use.

Several decades after an individual first suffers from this chain reaction, the very same diet that kicked off the process, acting along different pathways, will be the primary (but not the only) cause of the "diseases of civilization"—once again, diabetes, elevated blood fats, hypertension, excess weight and obesity, plus constipation with its consequences (varicose veins, varicocele, hemorrhoids, deep venous thrombosis, and diverticulitis). These diseases, many of them deadly, are nearly totally absent in ancient hunter populations and less industrialized societies today. Yet they are found in over half of the present-day adult population in Westernized societies. As chapter 7, "Origins: Food for Thought" explains, the clash between our genetically determined biology and the diet of Westernized societies is the decisive factor underlying all these diseases.

Modern dentistry can be justly proud of its achievements. More people are keeping more of their teeth longer than ever in modern times (Beltrán-Aguilar et al. 2005). However, we need to note that almost none of that improvement comes from dietary common sense in Westernized societies but from high-tech preventive and treatment measures. Community water fluoridation, in-office fluoride treatment, self-applied fluoride gels, and fluoride toothpastes (almost all toothpastes today) increase the resistance of teeth to decay. In-office application of pit and fissure sealants modifies tooth anatomy and close off the small gaps on tooth surfaces that trap bacteria and the degraded carbohydrates we feed them. Add to these the long list of dramatic restorative procedures at our disposal and we see the real reason for these advances. They are technological advances, not dietary ones. None will result in a decrease of the other chronic diseases of civilization.

Looking at it another way, North American modern dentistry, combined with better home care, has resulted in a 10 percent reduction in dental decay by the end of the twentieth century. Nearly 60 percent of children and adolescents ages six to nineteen have no fillings and no cavities today (Beltrán-Aguilar et al. 2005). But how does it stack up compared to decay incidence and prevalence in the pre-industrialized, pre-agricultural world? Then, almost no one had cavities. Similarly, then, almost no one suffered from the chronic diseases of civilization (Cockburn et al. 1998).

Consider the title of this chapter—Dental Decay: A Preventable Scourge. If dental decay and the chronic, systemic diseases of civilization are (mainly) caused by the same dietary factors, can we eliminate the latter with a diet that eliminates the former?

Bottom Line

1. Dental decay and chronic, systemic diseases (the diseases of civilization) share the same cause—a diet high in refined carbohydrates.
2. Dental decay in early life reliably predicts the arrival of these chronic systemic diseases in later life.
3. High-tech modern dentistry is rapidly lowering the rates of dental decay.
4. High-tech modern dentistry has no effect on the diseases of civilization. We can eliminate dental decay *and* chronic, systemic diseases (the diseases of civilization) from our lives and the lives of our children. All we need to do is align how we eat with how we were designed.

Chapter 9.

Your Gums, Your Heart

Coronary heart disease (CHD) is the world's number one killer. Ten risk factors have been identified, and the good news is that we have almost total control over seven of these. Here is the complete picture:

1. Age—not controllable
2. Gender—not controllable
3. Family history—not controllable
4. Excess weight/obesity—controllable
5. Elevated blood fats—controllable
6. Diabetes—controllable
7. Hypertension—controllable
8. Smoking—controllable
9. Lack of exercise—controllable
10. Inflammatory gum disease—controllable

We have no control over aging. Except for the diseases of childhood, the older we get the more likely we are to succumb to *most* diseases. A healthy old age is a myth. The best that we can do is to push the infirmities of old age as far down the road of life as possible. The proven way to do that is to align our habits with our design.

We also have no control over our gender. During their reproductive years, women have significant protection against CHD. On the whole, they develop CHD more than a decade later than men.

Family history is the last of the three risk factors that is beyond our control. Here too, women come off better. They are less affected by a negative family history.

All seven of the remaining CHD risk factors are within our control. Smoking and exercising are obviously in our control. But are diabetes, elevated blood fats, hypertension, and excess weight/obesity really controllable? Consider that all were exceptionally rare until modern times. In addition, they remain exceptionally rare in the few societies whose diets are still in line with our design. We can control them all if we hunt and gather at the grocery store.

All other chapters in this section deal with the major contribution of dietary refined carbohydrates to dental decay *plus* a long list of other chronic diseases that manifest themselves later in life, often decades later. These chapters look at how dental decay, easily diagnosed early by professionals, predictably shares its origins with the other chronic diseases that show up in later life.

In this chapter, we'll examine the inflammatory gum disease–heart disease connection (Cronin 2009), which is unrelated to refined carbohydrate consumption. North American dentists often find inflammatory gum disease in patients who have no dental decay, primarily because they come from cultures in which refined carbohydrates are not on the menu, much, yet. With globalization, we have seen the end of distance in the last generation, and major North American cities have large populations from other parts of the world. We see patients who have recently arrived from India, Pakistan, China, and other countries which have not, at this time, heartily embraced the processed foods and drinks that are so much a part of the destructive diet of Western nations.

While much of *Your Mouth, Your Health* deals with the connection between tooth decay and chronic disease, including hypertension and related heart disease, diabetes, elevated blood fats, excess weight/obesity, varicose veins, hemorrhoids, diverticulitis, and more, there is another mouth source that contributes to heart disease: gum inflammation, the most common form of gum disease.

Any medical term ending in "itis" refers to inflammation (pulpitis is inflammation of the tooth pulp (nerve), hepatitis is inflammation of the liver, tonsillitis is inflammation of the tonsils, arthritis is inflammation of the joints, colitis is inflammation of the colon, meningitis is inflammation of the meninges, tendonitis is inflammation of the tendons, encephalitis is inflammation of the brain, and so forth). Gum inflammation is called periodontitis.

A decade ago, scientists started looking for a relationship between periodontal disease and coronary artery disease. That connection has now been positively established and, in fact, today, the standard for all patients about to undergo heart surgery of any sort is to have a dental checkup and have their mouth cleaned up so that it is spotless (Abou-Raya et al. 2002).

Additionally, many studies establish the connection between heart disease and periodontitis, the most common form of inflammatory gum disease. One respected, large, and comprehensive investigation followed 9,760 individuals over a fourteen-year period to conclude that inflammatory gum disease is connected to an increased risk of heart disease (Mattila 1993). Dentists assess the extent of inflammatory gum disease by various methods. Commonly, we start with a screening to get a quick look at a person's general gum health. Studies show that correct screening—testing in the area of a small number of specifically selected teeth or selected areas of the mouth—is a good indication of the health of the gums in the whole mouth. Testing these subsets is fast and easy.

During screening, we test for gum health by assessing the color, texture, and appearance of the gums, checking pocket depth (how far we can gently push a special probe between a tooth and the gum), degree of bleeding on probing, and tooth mobility. We use particular X-ray views to see bone levels surrounding each tooth. If there is cause for concern, then we do a more detailed examination. Here, we typically use the same parameters, but we examine six locations for *each* tooth (Löe 1967). A shallow pocket depth, typically 2 mm or less, with no associated bleeding is considered to be one sign of gum health. However, many people with gum bleeding that they are able to ignore have a lot of pocketing in excess of 6 mm around many of their teeth.

If the inside of each pocket surrounding each tooth is lined with inflamed tissue, a common situation, the total area can add up to the size of the palm of your hand. You'd run to the doctor if you had that large an area of bleeding and inflammation anywhere on your skin. When it involves the gums, the skin of the jaws really, this bleeding takes place on the inner aspect of the pockets and not on the visible, outside aspect. Much of the time there are no perceptible signs to serve as warning signals. It's an easy matter to ignore.

It is important here to make a distinction between acute and chronic inflammation. Acute inflammation is our friend. It is a healing response to mechanical injury or some other physical insult like a burn, chemical irritation, infection by microorganisms, and so on. This healing response is characterized by five features: pain, redness, swelling, heat, and impaired function. Think of the last time you fell and skinned your knee. With the possible exception of the increased heat to the area, you could see all these features immediately after the fall. The right kind of thermometer could have shown you the increased heat too.

If the events that induced this healing response are not eliminated or overcome by the healing response and the inflammation lingers on, it becomes chronic. Chronic inflammation is *not* our friend. The acute inflammation defense cells begin to be replaced by other types of cells and tissue destruction and tissue healing takes place concurrently. Over time, the destruction wins if the condition is not treated or not treatable.

The definitive distinction between acute and chronic pain is based on patient history and a cellular-level microscopic analysis. The five features of acute inflammation are present in various degrees, but pain may be totally absent. For example, the pain of acute pulpitis can be excruciating but dentists commonly detect longstanding chronic pulpitis (usually on X-rays) that patients are completely unaware of. Periodontitis, a chronic disease, is painless.

Chronic hepatitis is rarely associated with pain. There are other examples.

Science is gaining better understanding of this complex phenomenon, to the extent that a vaccine will someday provide protection against periodontitis (Beevi et al. 2009).

At this point, it is known that chronic gum inflammation, that is, periodontitis, is one of the risk factors for heart disease (Beck et al. 1998) (Oe et al. 2009).

In much of the world, inflammatory gum disease happens *without* much of a dietary presence of refined carbohydrates. A diet devoid of refined carbohydrates can virtually guarantee tooth health, total absence of dental decay, and the near elimination of the chronic diseases we deal with in this book, but it is no guarantee of gum health.

Regular dental checkups and professional cleaning combined with appropriate antimicrobials can easily control gum inflammation. Dentists tailor individual patient cleaning frequency to meet individual patient needs. That frequency is an attribute of an individual's biology and not of the individual's dental insurance plan. In our office, we have people we call back once every *five years*, people we call back once every *two weeks*, and patients whose checkup frequency runs the entire gamut of frequencies in between. If you have any bleeding when you brush and floss, your dental checkups and professional cleanings are not frequent enough. You should see your dentist for a comprehensive examination, diagnosis, and treatment. Combined with a proper diet, you can eliminate two major risk factors (inflammatory gum disease and the refined carbohydrate causes of dental decay) and improve your heart health.

Bottom Line

1. We have full control over seven of the ten coronary heart disease risk factors.
2. Inflammatory gum disease is one of these risk factors.
3. Inflammatory gum disease is both very common and easily manageable in its early stages.

4. Your dentist can help you manage inflammatory gum disease even if it has progressed to later stages.
5. For each of us, there is an appropriate time span between dental hygiene visits.
6. Your dentist can teach you to improve your home care and, thus, safely decrease the frequency of your dental hygiene visits.

Chapter 10.

The Deadly Quartet Part 1: Excess Weight and Obesity

I use the term "the deadly quartet" for impact. It is an older term that health care professionals have now replaced with the less suggestive expression "the metabolic syndrome"—a cluster of signs and symptoms that characterize one disease (Vancheri Burgio, and Dovico).

Deadly Quartet Background

For more than fifty years now, scientists have debated two theories about the mouth health–systemic health connection. The first of these aligns with *Your Mouth, Your Health: Stop and Reverse Aging.* It states that excessive dietary refined carbohydrates (mainly sugar and white flour) lead to tooth decay early in life and, several decades later, to the other diseases we deal with here, including the deadly quartet:

1) Excess weight and obesity
2) Elevated blood fats
3) Diabetes
4) Hypertension

The deadly quartet's result is heart disease. In other words, dental decay is the early warning system, the proverbial "canary in the coalmine," for the arrival of the other diseases. Limiting dietary refined carbohydrates prevents them all.

In the mid-twentieth century, Thomas Cleave and John Yudkin, two scientists with medical backgrounds, formulated this theory by observing diseases of Africans living under tribal condition to those of their siblings and cousins who had moved to cities and went from eating from nature's pantry to eating refined carbohydrates (Yudkin 1965). All diseases we discuss in this book were nearly absent among Africans living under tribal conditions and common among their city-dwelling kin whose diets were high in refined carbs (Cleave 1975). Indeed, many trained observers have noted the absence of these diseases in all people living on unrefined foods—in other words, eating from nature's pantry.

The other theory, which Ancel Keys, who was equally qualified, proposed and supported, claims that excessive dietary fats are responsible for the deadly quartet. To prevent this deadly combination, Keys recommended a diet high in carbohydrates, either refined or not (Keys 1965) (Grande and Keys 1965). He stated correctly that dental decay arising from refined carbohydrates could be controlled by good mouth hygiene, fluorides, fissure sealants, antibacterial preparations, and fillings and crowns, each a form of the high-tech dentistry described in detail in chapter 8, "Dental Decay: The Preventable Scourge." Keys did not recognize the forecasting reliability of early-life tooth decay.

Researchers have now thoroughly tested both theories in well-designed clinical trials (Hujoel 2009). The scientific community currently widely accepts the Cleave–Yudkin theory.

As *Your Mouth, Your Health: Stop and Reverse Aging* has pointed out, according to this theory, we are exquisitely engineered for survival under conditions of constant food scarcity. Increasingly, abundance and, more importantly, an abundance of engineered, degraded food (primarily refined carbohydrates and engineered fats) is replacing scarcity. When our exquisitely engineered design collides with food exquisitely engineered for Big Food profit, Big

Food wins. Profitability trumps health. Engineered, degraded food abuses our exquisite design.

Excess Weight and Obesity

In the past decade, the number of overweight children has doubled in North America, and 60 percent of the population is overweight. In nature, there are no overweight animals. We are a part of nature. The good news is that most of us can be at the optimal weight range for our height and stay there. We simply need to align our diet and our lifestyles with our design. Simply does not mean easily. *Your Mouth, Your Health* is intended as a guide to understanding the dietary forces that we need to control in order to take charge of our health.

What are the benefits of maintaining optimal weight? The respected medical journal *The Lancet* recently published a study on the weight/life span data on close to one million people—a figure that would impress any biostatistician. *The Lancet* study concluded that people of normal weight can add three years to their lives compared to the moderately obese and a whole decade compared to the severely obese (Whitlock et al. 2009). Additionally, many other respected studies show that a higher quality of life is a part of being of normal weight (Lubetkin and Jia 2009) (Zahran et al. 2005).

As it does for all the diseases of civilization we review here, a diet high in refined carbohydrates in early life lays the groundwork for excess weight in later life. Dental decay appears first. Excess weight becomes visible next, often in the early teens, and is the easiest of all to notice. The others predictably follow.

The Math

When it comes to weight, our body understands grade school arithmetic only. If calories in exceed calories out, we gain weight. If calories out exceed calories in, we lose weight. To maintain weight, calories in must equal calories out. We can't get around the simple math. This simple formula explains why all weight loss diets work and why the results are almost always temporary—as we follow the diet and eliminate the calories we take in, we lose weight, and when the diet is over and our calorie intake increases, we gain it back.

To make the result permanent, we need to change our lifestyle.

If weight control is so simple, then why are we experiencing an epidemic of weight problems? Over 65 percent of North Americans are overweight, and over 30 percent are obese (Flegal et al. 2002)! North Americans, much like the rest of the developed world, obsess over weight-loss diets. An Internet search for any of the key words *diet, weight control, obesity,* and the like produces tens of millions of hits.

Why Is Western Society Fat?

For the answer to this vexing question, we need to look into three issues:

1. Genetics or heredity
2. Consumption of debased, Big Food products
3. Lifestyle aided and abetted by Big Food

Heredity

Heredity is the easiest "cause" of excess weight to understand, so we will get it out of the way first.

What if our genes are making us fat (Dedoussis et al. 2007)? After all, both of our parents are fat. We can't help it.

Hereditary defects arise less than five times in one thousand births (Dykes et al. 1953). That's less than 0.5 percent! Over 65 percent of the North American population is overweight. No, most of us cannot blame heredity.

But what about diabetes? It runs in the family.

Excess weight and obesity are not due to diabetes; nor is diabetes a result of excess weight and obesity. Neither is dental decay due to diabetes or excess weight and obesity. All three have the same main cause.[18] The decay predicts the excess weight and obesity, just

18 While most diseases, in fact, have more than one cause (they are said to be multifactorial), in most cases, there is one single, overwhelmingly important cause. Eliminate that one and the rest hardly matter. By

like it predicts the diabetes and just like it predicts the diseases of civilization. The abundance of cheap, engineered, degraded food is the major contributing factor to all the conditions.

Consumption of Debased, Big Food Products

In nature during periods of food abundance, all animals increase the size of their populations, not the size of their bodies. We human animals do exactly the same, unless we are surrounded at every turn by cheap, engineered, highly palatable food, concocted to be nearly addictive and pushed by in-your-face marketing pressure. The few remaining hunter and gatherer societies on the planet demonstrate that absent these factors, human populations do not increase their individual weight during periods of abundance. The Cleave–Yudkin hypothesis has constantly withstood careful scrutiny.

No nation in history has successfully reversed an epidemic of excess weight and obesity. Japan, not a country in which excess weight is a notable problem, is the first country to have taken official steps to prevent it, having studied the soaring costs of excess weight in other countries (Onishi 2008). Japan recently enacted a law that requires companies and local governments to monitor the waistlines of middle-aged Japanese people and to target explicit goals. Companies and local governments that fail to reach these goals are fined. In the North American context, such a law would be political suicide. No policymaker will ever propose it; Big Food will continue to increase both North America's waistlines and its bottom lines.

In our own lives, however, each of us can prevent or reverse excess weight. Many have done it. We have to be aware that our bodies are not wrongly built but we can wrongly use them.

How does consuming an abundance of engineered, degraded food—primarily refined carbohydrates and engineered fats—abuse the way we were designed? To repeat information covered in chapter 2, processing carbohydrates alters them in two major ways. First,

---

avoiding refined carbohydrates, mainly sugar and white flour, we can virtually eliminate diseases of civilization.

it removes the carb's fiber and micronutrients, and second, it concentrates its sugar. The second is, in part, a result of the first. Removing fiber leads to sugar concentration. Our evolved hunger–satiety response is unable to deal with the alteration in a normal manner, and we overeat.

Keeping that in mind, let us compare 100 mg of fresh, chopped carrots (one cup) to an equal weight of typical, commercially made carrot cake.[19]

1. With the fresh carrots, 40 calories and 5 gm of sugar are carried through the digestive system by 3 gm of fiber.
2. With the carrot cake, 296 calories and 25 gm of sugar are carried through the digestive system by 1 gm of fiber. Sugar is a highly refined carbohydrate.

Note that we are looking at equal portion sizes here with a 740 percent difference in caloric content (Divide 296 by 40 to get 7.4, or 740 percent)!

Chapter 14, "Constipation and Its Consequences" shows that when we digest the fresh carrots, aided by the fiber, the 40 calories move quickly from entrance to exit, and our bodies absorb only a part of the already small caloric content. Chapter 12, "Diabetes," shows that during digestion of natural, unrefined carbohydrates, blood sugar rises slowly and then drops at a rate determined by the effectiveness of the body's insulin production and/or insulin use.

When digesting the carrot cake, the more than seven times greater caloric content (largely because of fat), with a fraction of the fiber, moves slowly along the intestinal tract, and our bodies absorb a higher percentage of the caloric content. Digesting the carrot cake abuses the way we were designed. There are no refined carbohydrates in nature.[20]

---

19 Commercially made carrot cake includes fat and salt which, with the sugar, add up to the irresistible, terrible trio we discussed in chapter 6, "Vitamins and Minerals."
20 Honey comes close, but it was rarely on the menu of our hunter–gatherer ancestors.

Lifestyle

Each and every one of the thousands of weight-reduction diets works—in the short run. For the enduring and permanent ideal weight, dieters need a lifestyle change.

Bottom Line

1. Our body understands grade school arithmetic only. To lose weight, we need to reduce our caloric intake and/or increase our caloric burn rate until we reach our goal.
2. Once we get there, we need to adopt a lifestyle whereby our caloric intake equals our caloric burn rate.

Chapter 11.

The Deadly Quartet Part 2: Elevated Blood Fats

For practical purposes, there are only three things we need to know about elevated blood fats:

1. Elevated blood fats are a part of the deadly quartet (along with excess weight, pre-diabetes or full-blown diabetes, and hypertension with associated heart disease). These four can occur in isolation but rarely do so.
2. Eating the way we were designed to eat prevents elevated blood fats or reverses them if they are established.
3. There are no symptoms connected to elevated blood fats that suggest there is trouble ahead. That is, those who have elevated blood fats don't know it. Only specific blood tests can detect elevated blood fats.

You might impress the cocktail party circuit by throwing around ten-dollar words like hyperlipidemia, dyslipidemia, hypercholesterolemia, and hypertriglyceridemia, but unless you are a physician or a nutrition scientist, the three points above are all you need to know for best possible health. In dentistry, we pay attention to elevated blood fats mainly because some of the drugs used to control them can interact with some of the drugs we use.

If you have come this far in this book, you know that dental decay in early life accurately predicts elevated blood fats in later life, unless the decay-causing diet ends soon enough.

How soon is soon enough? Adopting a healthy lifestyle, including eating right, never happens too soon. Let's take a look at cholesterol, one of the blood fats. It is common knowledge that cholesterol is an essential structural part of cells, as well as being an important component of some hormones and vitamins. We can't do without it. It is also common knowledge that too much cholesterol in the blood stream can build up on artery walls leading to atherosclerosis. That can constrict arteries to the point that blood flow can stop entirely. A heart attack or a stroke can follow. Each can be incapacitating or even fatal.

Autopsies performed on soldiers killed in action during the Korean War some sixty years ago showed that over 75 percent had the beginnings of atherosclerosis, in other words, cholesterol deposits on their artery walls. These young Americans were in their twenties and early thirties! Long before enlisting, they ate a lot of refined carbohydrates, mainly sugar and white flour, the prominent features of debased, engineered Big Food products (Joseph et al. 1993). To be fair, smoking, another important factor in heart disease, was common at the time.

A decade later, the same study reported on autopsies performed on Vietnam War fatalities. It showed that only 45 percent of the young casualties had atherosclerosis. An encouraging step in the right direction, nonetheless, it is very far away from the 0 percent rate among people getting their food from Mother Nature's pantry.

But doesn't it seem logical that high levels of dietary fats would lead to high levels of blood fats? A review of chapter 10, "Excess Weight and Obesity," will remind us that Ancel Keys did claim exactly that. Keys recommended a diet high in carbohydrates, refined or not, to prevent elevated blood fats.

His theory had a lot of support for a while but was eventually sidelined by compelling studies that showed that high levels of dietary refined carbohydrates are central to elevated blood fats (Hofmann and Tschöp 2009) (Perona et al. 2009). Survey after survey, for instance, showed that the traditional, very high-fat diet of Arctic people actually protected them from cardiovascular disease. These studies examined large numbers of Quebec Inuit; native Greenlanders (Bang et al. 1980); and the Sámis of Finland, Norway, Russia, and Sweden (Luoma et al. 1995). Among these populations, the mortality rate from heart disease was low (Bjerregaard, Mulvad, and Pedersen 1997) (Dyerberg and Hjorne 1975). It is noteworthy that the Arctic people's traditional dietary fats came from marine sources, which have high levels of omega-3 fatty acids and no saturated fats. (For a discussion of fatty acids and saturated fats, see chapter 4, "Fats: Love Them, You Can't Leave Them.") Equally noteworthy and not surprising for readers of this book, as these Arctic people began to drift away from their traditional diets and adopt Western diets high in refined carbohydrates, their incidence of heart disease began to increase in direct proportion (Bersamin et al. 2008) (Sharma et al. 2009).

Indeed, that 0 percent rate of atherosclerosis caused by elevated blood fats is a realistic goal for anyone. As we saw earlier, with the right diet—one approximating our ancestral diet—all chronic diseases of civilization are preventable, stoppable, and reversible. That includes high blood fats, which lead to atherosclerosis and are one aspect of the deadly quartet.

Bottom Line

1. Elevated blood fats are one aspect of the deadly quartet (metabolic syndrome). The others are excess weight, pre-diabetes or full-blown diabetes, and hypertension with associated heart disease. These four can occur in isolation but do so rarely.

2. There are no symptoms of elevated blood fats. Those who have the problem don't know they have the problem. Physicians diagnose elevated blood fats by looking for signs that show up in specific blood tests.

3. Eating the way we were designed to eat prevents elevated blood fats or reverses them if they are established.

Chapter 12.

The Deadly Quartet Part 3: Diabetes

Almost anyone can avoid, delay, or reduce the impact of diabetes by understanding this chapter and following its recommendations. Diabetes here refers to what the health professionals call type 2 diabetes. It accounts for about 90 percent of all cases. Type 1 diabetes and gestational diabetes [21] make up the others. They cannot be prevented (yet) and need an ongoing, physician-monitored approach to treatment. Understanding this chapter and following its recommendations will diminish the brunt of these forms of diabetes as well (Gross, Ford, and Liu 2004).

What is diabetes? Diabetes is a grouping of several diseases that show high levels of blood sugar (glucose) either because of defective insulin production or defective insulin use by the

---

21 **Type 1 diabetes**, previously called juvenile-onset diabetes, affects young people. Sufferers' pancreases do not make insulin, the hormone responsible for glucose metabolism. People with type 1 diabetes must take insulin for life.

Type 2 diabetes, previously called adult-onset diabetes, starts in later life. The pancreas makes insulin, but the tissues that use it in glucose metabolism become increasingly resistant or intolerant to it over time when refined carbohydrate consumption is high.

Gestational diabetes is similar to type 2 diabetes. It needs treatment to avoid complications for the baby.

cells of the body or both. It was an early death sentence prior to the discovery of insulin by Canadian researchers Sir Frederick Banting and Dr. Charles Best.

Insulin is a hormone manufactured by the pancreas. Its primary function is to direct the body's use of glucose to meet immediate energy needs as well as future energy needs by storing blood sugar in the liver, muscle cells, and fat cells. In defective insulin production or defective insulin use by the cells of the body, much of the glucose derived from our food stays in the bloodstream aimlessly, with little direction.

What causes diabetes? Being this far along in the book, we know the main cause in most cases—a diet high in refined carbohydrates.

Overall, about 8 percent of the total population has type 2 diabetes, more than half of it undiagnosed. That includes children, adolescents and adults (Murtaugh et al. 2003). Almost all of these cases are self-inflicted and preventable (Kopp 2003).

In dentistry, we take special precautions for our diabetic patients (Tekavec 2009). In these patients, gum disease is more common and more difficult to treat. Their overall healing capacity is diminished.

Other diabetic complications are blindness, kidney damage, heart disease, and lower-limb amputations. All of these can be eased by controlling:

1) Blood glucose levels
2) Blood fat levels
3) Hypertension
4) Excess weight

Just like dental decay, each is virtually absent in today's hunter–gatherer societies and populations or individuals that still eat from Mother Nature's pantry. Again, dental decay does not cause these conditions, rather, all are caused by the same diet—a diet high in refined carbohydrates. Decay predicts them. Each could be absent from the lives of any of us if we hunt and gather in the grocery store and look for foods from Mother Nature's pantry (Murtaugh et al. 2003) (Tabatabai and Li 2000) (Venn and Mann 2004).

How does a diet high in refined carbohydrates cause type 2 diabetes? Think of what gentle waves lapping at a dock do to it over extended time. Then compare that to what repeated pounding by huge waves does to the dock.

Let's look at the physiologic parallel. When any animal eats, some of the macronutrients in the food, aided by the micronutrients (see chapters 1 through 6), get converted to glucose. Under Mother Nature's conditions, operating in harmony with how we are wired, our bodies convert unprocessed food to blood sugar slowly and the glucose gets into the bloodstream slowly. The concentration of blood sugar rises to a peak gently, and then insulin converts it to energy or to fat or prepares it for storage in the liver and muscle for later use. These are the gentle waves lapping at the dock.

On the other hand, we convert highly processed (refined) carbohydrates—mainly sugar and including dietary glucose itself, white flour, and white rice—into blood sugar quickly and the glucose gets into the bloodstream quickly. The concentration of blood sugar rises to a peak quickly and then drops at a rate determined by the effectiveness of the body's insulin production and/or insulin use. This is the repeated pounding of the dock by huge waves.

Both are cyclic phenomena. Gentle, shallow cycles do little damage; intense, steep cycles do serious damage (Thorburn et al 1987).

For example, when we eat potatoes, our bodies convert the starch in the potatoes into sugar, and this sugar is absorbed into the bloodstream in a slow, gentle fashion. On the other hand, when we drink pop or eat highly sugared breakfast cereal with a low fiber content, we are looking at a physiologically violent process. Without the modifying effect of fiber, sugar gets into the blood stream quickly with brutal and unhealthy demands on our metabolic activity.

Automobile wear and tear is another good analogy. Driven at highway speeds for extended periods, a vehicle lasts a lot longer than it would if it were constantly driven in a stop-and-go fashion. The effect of a diet high in refined carbohydrates (the common Western, debased-food diet) is like that of stop-and-go driving. The vehicle, be it a car or a human body, gets destroyed faster.

What are the early signs and symptoms[22] of diabetes? They are a combination of lethargy, mental fatigue, frequent urination, and increased thirst. Now, all of us experience these four signs and symptoms from time to time, and each of them can arise on its own for reasons unrelated to diabetes. But when they appear together and become frequent, it is time to see the doctor.

After developing full-blown diabetes, people age physiologically at twice their chronologic rate of aging. For example, people who get diabetes at age thirty are fifty years old physiologically by age forty. All debilitating conditions that are a part of normal aging develop sooner. Death comes sooner.

Bottom Line

1. Type 2 diabetes makes up about 90 percent of all cases. Type 1 diabetes, gestational diabetes, and some other types make up the other 10 percent.
2. By following the common sense, well-established dietary recommendations in this book, you can prevent, delay, or reverse type 2 diabetes.
3. Following these guidelines also renders type 1 diabetes, gestational diabetes, and the other types easier to manage.
4. Type 2 diabetes was almost unknown in the Western world before the twentieth century.

---

22 Signs are visible to others. Examples in the case of diabetes are frequent urination, as well as many direct and indirect lab tests. On the other hand, only the patient is aware of symptoms. Examples for diabetes are lethargy, mental fatigue, and increased thirst.

In countries that are adopting Westernized ways of eating, type 2 diabetes among the young, as well as in adults, is reaching epidemic proportions in parallel with the increase in sugar consumption. Authorities in all these countries are aware of it. None have reversed it.

We knew in the sixties that executives of cigarette companies did not smoke. Do Big Food executives today feed junk food cereals to their children?

5. Type 2 diabetes is virtually absent in today's hunter–gatherer societies and in populations and individuals who eat from Mother Nature's pantry. It can be absent from any of our lives.

6. In the Western world, the incidence and prevalence of type 2 diabetes are rising exponentially and in parallel with the rise in refined carbohydrate consumption.

7. Dental decay early in life is a reliable predictor of type 2 diabetes and its consequences in later life.

8. While no country in history has ever reversed the rise of type 2 diabetes and its consequences, we can reverse, prevent, and eliminate it our own lives.

9. The reasonable and established dietary recommendations in this book provide the simple, effective, and pleasant answer.

10. Good, unbiased sources of information about managing diabetes can be found at www.nia.nih.gov/, www.diabetes.niddk.nih.gov/, and http://www.diabetes.ca/.

Chapter 13.

The Deadly Quartet Part 4: Hypertension and Heart Disease

Hypertension is called the silent killer. It's silent because, like with high blood fats, there are no symptoms. It's a killer because, like high blood fats, it leads to deadly heart disease. Heart disease is the leading cause of death in the developed world (Anderson et al. 2000). Because of its importance in mortality and morbidity, scientists have sought to understand the connected causes for many decades now. As with most scientific endeavors, "the truth" changes on a regular basis. Scientists have uncovered the simple, causal connections between heart disease and its causes. But researchers must do a lot more digging to uncover new truths.

Because numerous macronutrient and micronutrient studies have shown no promising findings that connect the nutrients to hypertension and heart disease, it is clear that researchers need to study the whole diet instead of its parts.

It is sobering to note that heart disease was rare in *all* hunter–gatherer societies that medical anthropologists ever studied (Kopp 2003) (Eaton 2006). These were societies with no access to modern health care. Further, study after study shows that hypertension and heart disease remain rare today among people following traditional lifestyles (Pavan et al. 1999). These are simple, causal connections.

Other studies, equally compelling, show that when people move from traditional-diet societies to Western-diet societies, they experience a remarkable rise in hypertension and heart disease rates. The Bedouin of Southern Israel (Abu-Saad et al. 2001), the blacks of South Africa (Vorster 2002), Australian Aborigines (O'Dea, Spargo, and Nestel 1982), the Japanese of Japan compared to the Japanese of America (Kitamura et al. 2009), all show the unmistakable connection between heart health and eating from Mother Nature's pantry and, conversely, heart disease and eating from Big Food's pantry. Of course, since we have read this far, we know that eating from Mother Nature's panty protects against *all* the diseases we discuss in this book, while eating from Big Food's pantry promotes them. Dental decay predicts them all.

Respected health organizations, such as the American Heart Association, recognize these connections. Excessive consumption of refined carbohydrates, primarily sugars, combined with engineered fats, is central to the diseases of civilization.

In chapter 9, "Your Gums, Your Heart," we discussed the ten risk factors of heart disease. As a reminder, here they are again:

1. Age—not controllable
2. Gender—not controllable
3. Family history—not controllable
4. Excess weight/obesity—controllable
5. Elevated blood fats—controllable
6. Diabetes—controllable
7. Hypertension—controllable
8. Smoking—controllable
9. Lack of exercise—controllable
10. Inflammatory gum disease—controllable

Let's now look at hypertension, the last of the deadly quartet. We will review current recommendations, each based on the latest evidence. With the possible exception of inflammatory gum disease, which we looked into in chapter 9, all of the risk factors described above are familiar territory. Inflammatory gum disease has come under the microscope only recently and is just beginning to reach the general public.

Impartial scholarly research repeatedly confirms that eating from Mother Nature's pantry lowers the incidence of hypertension and heart disease. In southern Europe, fruits, vegetables, legumes, grains, fish, and chicken make up the dietary foundation, and olive oil is the main source of fat; hypertension and heart disease rates are low. The dietary choices are the basis of the well-known and well-publicized Mediterranean Diet (Ness and Powles 1997) (McKeown et al. 2009).

Hypertension and heart disease rates also used to be low in Asia. The traditional Asian diet is similar to the Mediterranean diet with two modifications. Rice takes the place of wheat, and peanut oil takes the place of olive oil; both oils are benign monounsaturated fats. Neither the Mediterranean nor the Asian diet is low in fats. Rather, they are low in saturated fats; their main sources of fat are olive oil, peanut oil, fish, nuts, seeds, and certain vegetable oils. By contrast, in northern Europe and North America where processed foods, primarily sugar, combined with red meat, cheese, and other sources of saturated fats are common, hypertension and heart disease are epidemic (Hu et al. 2000).

A Word about Sodium

We have known for a long time that the body needs a balance between sodium and potassium intake to function normally. Medical researchers have solidly established the connection between excessive levels of dietary sodium and hypertension. That needed sodium–potassium equilibrium is simply not possible in the context of the dietary choices in Western countries, where daily sodium consumption is three times higher than that of potassium.

Table salt, sodium chloride, is the main source of sodium in the Western diet, while baking soda and MSG are minor sources. Big Food relies heavily on the terrible trio of salt, fat, and sugar to make its packaged foods palatable and easier to sell. Home cooking is the only reliable way to bring the sodium–potassium equilibrium into alignment. Replace the sodium chloride in all the salt shakers with potassium chloride, and use it in cooking. Potassium chloride is a safer alternative.

A Word about Exercise

Sales of exercise equipment and gym memberships are on the rise, in parallel with the rise in excess weight and obesity. It almost seems that the former is causing the latter. Of course, that is not the case, but we need surprisingly little exercise for optimal heart health and health in general. A fifteen-minute walk five times a week reduces the risk of heart attack death by nearly 50 percent! Combine exercise with eating from Mother Nature's pantry, and we can reduce that risk almost entirely.

A Word about Stress

The fight-or-flight response to challenges that is a part of our genetic heritage is inappropriate in modern life. It is another example of the continuous dissonance between our genome and our environment. With no socially acceptable way to channel the hormonal setup that leads to fight or flight, we get stressed. Stress in modern life is practically a constant.

Practicing Benson's relaxation response twice a day—breathing deeply and regularly with your eyes closed, your muscles relaxed, and your thoughts banished, in a quiet place—is a documented and effective technique (Benson and Herbert 1983). So are yoga, midday naps, prayer, and meditation—the list of effective stress busters is long. Look into them.

Any of these techniques is more enjoyable and less costly than the current, all-too-familiar "treatments" sweeping the Western world. While no evidence-based studies show that these methods— angioplasty, coronary artery bypass surgery, or drug-coated stents— prevent heart attacks or death for most patients, the costs are clear: more than $60 billion a year in North America. We in North America don't need to be among the victims; we can be like the people eating traditional choices. The choice is ours.

Bottom Line

1. Don't allow yourself to carry excess weight.
2. If you are overweight, get to your right weight and stay there.
3. Get your blood fats and pre-diabetes or full-blown type 2 diabetes under control. Consult your physician on this.
4. Get a minimum of fifteen minutes of moderate exercise five times each week.
5. Dump the sodium chloride from your saltshaker and fill it with potassium chloride.
6. If you smoke, seek a cessation method that will work for you. Resources that will help you curb this devastating addiction are at your fingertips. Start with a simple Internet search for "smoking cessation programs."
7. See your dentist to ensure and maintain your gum health.
8. Hunt and gather from Nature's Pantry in the grocery store.

Chapter 14.

Constipation and Its Consequences: Varicose Veins, Varicocele, Hemorrhoids, Deep Venous Thrombosis, Diverticulitis, and Yes, Excess Weight

In the carbohydrates chapter, we pointed out that processing (degrading) removes about 90 percent of the sugar beet or sugar cane to get table sugar and about 30 percent of wheat and rice to get white flour and white rice. Let's now take a look at how this degrading of carbohydrates affects the gastrointestinal (GI) tract.

What do "refiners" remove? Physically, most of the material processing removes is fiber. Fiber and its fruit equivalent, pectin, are not nutrients. Their role is more biophysical than biochemical. There are no deficiency diseases resulting from fiber removal, such as we see when we don't consume enough of the essential nutrients. Vitamin C deficiency results in scurvy; iodine deficiency leads to goiter; thiamin deficiency leads to beriberi, a nervous system disease that leads to lethargy and fatigue and a host of other complications; and a lack of protein is connected with kwashiorkor, the acute type of malnutrition characterized by distended bellies and severe edema. As a result, fiber and pectin were among the last food components to receive the attention of science.

But when fiber and pectin began to get serious consideration, their role in the function of the GI tract became increasingly clear. Fiber and pectin influence the absorption of nutrients, calories, and water, as well as the composition and quantity of the stool by speeding up transit time. Variously called orofaecal transit time, whole gut transit time, orocaecal transit time—not the subject of polite conversation—transit time refers to the length of time food needs to pass from the entrance (the mouth) to the exit (the anus). People primarily eating foods as Mother Nature presents them to us have a transit time that is less than half of that found among people primarily eating the debased foods of the Western, industrialized diet. Natural transit time results in a daily bowel movement. The output is nearly odorless. Compare that to the twice weekly bowel movement so common with people who eat a primarily Western, industrialized diet—a twenty-four-hour event versus one of forty-eight to ninety-six hours! Let's not talk about odor.

Mother Nature's diet, the hunter–gatherer diet, supplies 30 mg or more of fiber and pectin daily; the Western, industrialized diet supplies about half of that. The relationship between dietary fiber and pectin and transit time is a direct one. The dramatic difference has dramatic health implications. The speed of that journey is critical, as slower transit time, colonic stasis, is a serious health hazard over time.

What happens as a result of stasis? Dental decay, the first disease of civilization to show up is, again, the early and reliable predictor of colonic stasis.

People whose diet approximates the hunter–gatherer diet, one with high levels of dietary fiber and pectin, show a notably lower risk for developing any of these (Cherbut et al. 1997).

To understand how stasis happens, we must examine stool formation. First, most of the water that we consume in addition to and with our food is removed for physiologic use as it gets closer to the exit. Stasis simply removes more water since the food spends more time in the part of the GI tract responsible for water removal. This results in hard, difficult to pass stool, or constipation. The consequences are varicose veins, varicoceles, hemorrhoids, deep venous thrombosis and diverticulitis.

Additionally, slower transit time allows the GI tract to remove more calories from food, resulting in greater caloric intake by the body.

Constipation

Constipation is a widespread and vexing problem that disrupts people's lives and places a huge and costly load both on individual patients and the health care system. Studies show that as many as 20 percent of the population suffers from constipation at one time or another. Laxative manufacturing is a billion-dollar industry.

Constipation is not a part of the normal aging process, although there is a greater prevalence among older people. This increase with age is because older people have lived on these debased foods for longer periods of time than have their younger counterparts and older people are not as active as they used to be. Decreased mobility contributes to constipation, as do many drugs that older populations use much more than do younger people (Spinzi et al. 2009).

Many treatment options for people with constipation are available with varying degrees of evidence to support their use. None can match the documented effectiveness of increasing fiber and pectin consumption, decreasing refined carb consumption, and throwing modest exercise into the mix. Fruits and vegetables plus walking or its equivalent, in other words, combine to make up nature's unequalled colonic flush.

Most treatment options outside this simple recommendation exist for economic reasons. Somebody wants to sell something.

Let's take a look at the consequences of constipation.

Varicose Veins

In the early 1940s, reviewing the medical records of over one hundred ten thousand South African Zulu patients living under tribal conditions (in other words, eating no refined carbohydrates), the British surgeon Thomas Cleave found *three* patients with varicose veins—*three* (Cleave 1974)! That's pretty close to 0 percent. His review included over three thousand pregnant women. Review the medical literature for the incidence and prevalence of varicose veins in industrialized societies today and you'll find nearly one thousand scholarly articles. These articles report a range of varicose veins prevalence—up to 56 percent in men and 60 percent in women—in the populations studied (Beebe-Dimmer et al. 2005).

Not surprisingly, the diets of the industrialized societies study subjects consist of heavy doses of debased food (Traber, Mazzolai, and Läuchli 2009). Varicose veins are almost entirely an environmental issue, and so whether or not we suffer from this ailment is entirely within our control (Sudoł-Szopińska, Błachowiak, and Koziński 2006).

Fiber removal, which is part of processing carbohydrates, slows transit time so that the body takes much of the water at the colon level. The stool becomes hard and loads the colon to a greater extent than it is designed for. The colon distends and presses on leg veins, which become partially blocked and distended. If that goes on long enough, varicose veins develop.

For anatomic reasons, varicose veins are more common in the left leg than the right. As the colon descends, it crosses over the left leg vein, which brings the blood up to the heart. The constipated colon is full of hard material so it obstructs that left leg blood flow, leading to left leg varicose veins more often than right leg varicose veins.

Varicocele

In men, an anatomic structure called the spermatic cord contains arteries, veins, nerves, and tubes, among other things. It circulates blood to and from the testicles. Varicose veins in this part of a man's anatomy are called varicocele. Caused by the same forces we described under the varicose veins heading above, varicocele is also usually found on the left side. About 10 to 15 percent of men and teenage boys are affected (Biyani, Cartledge, and Janetschek 2009). There appears to be no connection between varicocele and fertility or any other male dysfunction; nonetheless it can be uncomfortable. Health practitioners treat this condition with several types of safe and effective treatments (Soffer et al. 1983) (Evers, Collins, and Clarke 2009).

Like with varicose veins and all other conditions described in this book, an ounce of prevention is worth a pound of cure. Eating as we've recommend provides the simple, effective answer.

Hemorrhoids

By now, you're catching on. We are looking at another variation on the same theme, just in a different part of the anatomy. Hemorrhoids are varicose veins of the exit of the GI tract. Varicose veins, varicocele, and hemorrhoids result from chronically high bowel pressure, which in turn results from slow transit time, which results from eating the debased foods of the Western, industrialized diet. The high bowel pressure interferes with venous blood flow (Haas, Fox, and Haas 1984).

All of these conditions have many other contributing causes, incidentally. They are said to be multifactorial. The other contributing causes are minor by comparison, a clear conclusion when you consider that all of these conditions are virtually absent among people who live under tribal conditions and eat no refined carbohydrates. For the same reason, they were virtually absent from Western societies until the twentieth century. The other contributing causes were present all along but were insufficient to trigger these conditions. Dental decay in early life is a reliable predictor of their eventual arrival.

So, to eliminate these unpleasant conditions we can move in with the Zulus. Alternatively, we can stay put but change our diet from degraded food to real food—food the way Mother Nature gives it to us in the first place. She never heard of refined carbohydrates.

Deep Venous Thrombosis

A thrombus is a blood clot attached to a blood vessel wall. There are no thrombi in healthy blood vessels. When the thrombus breaks off from its blood vessel wall and starts to float downstream, it is called an embolism. If it originates in the deep leg veins it can travel to the lung arteries and plug them, leading to death. There is an increased incidence and prevalence of plugged lung arteries (pulmonary embolism) that perfectly parallels the ever-increasing presence of refined carbohydrates in Western, industrialized diets.

In the middle of the nineteenth century, the father of pathology, Rudolf Virchow, proposed three causes of deep venous thrombosis: venous stasis, damage to blood vessel walls, and changes in the blood (Esmon 2009). Today's physician still keeps these three in mind when making a diagnosis. Damage to blood vessel walls and changes in the blood are within limited personal control, but modern medicine can do a great deal to mitigate the pathology (Spencer et al. 2009). Happily, the elimination of venous stasis is within our complete control by the simple limitation of dietary refined carbohydrates. That alone is enough to eliminate deep venous thrombosis in most people.

Diverticulitis

Fiber-deficient, Western, industrialized diets result in chronic increased pressure inside the colon, which can lead to protrusions of the lining of the colon through the colon wall to form pouches. The condition is called diverticulosis and is the most common physical abnormality of the large bowel in the Western world (Floch and Bina 2004). About 60 percent of people sixty or over develop diverticulosis. When the pouches become inflamed, we have diverticulitis (Parra-Blanco 2006). About a quarter of people with diverticulosis develop diverticulitis which is potentially fatal (Pfeifer 2008).

Simple medical management is usually enough to treat the initial bouts of diverticulitis (Bahadursingh et al. 2003). If it recurs, then surgery is usually the next step (Hoffmann and Kruis 2005).

Like all other conditions we discuss in this book, diverticulosis and its derivative, diverticulitis, were almost unheard of before the twentieth century. They now constitute an increasing larger share of surgical and gastroenterological workload. Their incidence has been on a steady rise throughout the entire twentieth century and on.

These conditions are still almost unheard of in African countries, where people eat from Mother Nature's pantry. They could be almost unheard of in any of our lives. Dental decay early in life is a reliable predictor of diverticulosis development in later life.

Excess Weight

How does the dung beetle survive? There is enough nutrition including calories in dung to allow the nearly five thousand species of dung beetle to thrive. Faster transit times eliminate more calories and nutrients, leaving more for the beetle. There are so many calories in dung produced through fast transit time that, in some parts of the world, people have been using it as fuel for centuries (Winterhalder, Larsen, and Thomas 1974).

Practitioners of animal husbandry closely study the cost/benefit analysis of feed. Farmers study carcass composition and retail cuts yield associated with different feeding protocols. They need to get more for the finished animal than the cost of finishing it. Academic journals have published many studies dealing with nutrient intake minus nutrient elimination in farm animals. The economic motivation is powerful.

There are very few similar studies for human subjects. With people, studying nutrient intake alone is an economic motivator for Big Food. More looks better on Big Food financial statements; it is worse for the consumer.

Until more PhD candidates undertake comprehensive nutrient intake/nutrient elimination studies in human beings, we have to be content with the certainty that a faster transit time eliminates more calories than a slower transit time. The exact number of calories eliminated for specific foods is known for animal feed only.

If you are among the millions wrestling with weight issues, work on developing a taste for whole wheat and brown rice products while keeping your sugar consumption to about 5 percent of your daily caloric intake. With a few exceptions, that is Mother Nature's upper limit for sugar in fruits and vegetables.

Personally, I enjoy Italian and French restaurants where whole wheat bread is rarely on the menu. I bring my own.

Excess weight is not a consequence of constipation. However, both are caused, in part, by the same nutrient intake/nutrient elimination imbalance skewed by slow transit times. This imbalance contributes to excess weight in a noteworthy way. Its contribution to constipation is major.

How to Escape and Never Again be Plagued by Constipation and Its Consequences

Like we do with so many other sins, we breach the central commandment of this book—*thou shalt not refine carbohydrates*—more often than we observe it.

Happily, we can avoid this sin in our own lives.

No society in history has ever reversed the evils of disobeying this fundamental commandment. It is true that many diseases resulting from violating it are declining. For example, half the children entering high school in the Western world have no fillings and no cavities. The incidence and prevalence of heart disease are down. Diabetes is no longer the kiss of death, even though both its incidence and prevalence are on the rise. Medication and surgery are controlling, with varying degrees of success, elevated blood fats, hypertension, excess weight, obesity, kidney disease, memory decline, constipation, varicose veins, hemorrhoids, diverticulitis, and more.

But the central cause of these diseases, the refining of carbohydrates, remains in place. Any one of us can eliminate or control any and all of them by obeying this central commandment. And if we stray occasionally, it won't make much of a difference.

Bottom Line

1. Constipation and its consequences—varicose veins, varicocele, hemorrhoids, deep venous thrombosis, diverticulitis, and excess weight—were almost unknown in the Western world before the twentieth century.

2. Constipation and its consequences are practically non-existent today in populations that still live under tribal conditions and eat from Mother Nature's pantry.

3. Their incidence and prevalence are rising exponentially and parallel to the rise in refined carbohydrate consumption in the Western world.

4. Dental decay early in life is a reliable predictor of constipation and its consequences in later life.

5. No country in history has ever reversed the rise of excess weight and constipation with its consequences.

6. On a personal level, we can reverse, prevent, and eliminate excess weight and constipation with its consequences in our own lives.

7. The lifestyle recommendations in the last chapter of this book provide the simple, effective, and pleasant answer to avoiding these diseases and ailments.

Chapter 15.

The Only Guide to Eating
You'll Ever Need

Earlier, I promised to show that, contrary to common belief, potatoes are nutritionally better than apples. In fact, potatoes are so nutritious that they were the dietary staple of the great Inca civilization (Hodge 1951). No civilization was ever built on apples. With the addition of small amounts of fats and proteins, potatoes with their skin make for a nutritionally complete diet. We can't say that about apples, excellent though they be nutritionally. A glance at any of the many nutrition data Web sites shows that to be true. (Nutrition Data: Know What You Eat, located at www.nutritiondata.com is an excellent resource.)

In the mid-eighteenth century, the population of Ireland exploded to eight million, soon after potatoes from South America became a part of the diet. Conversely, about one hundred years later, the failure of the Irish potato crop resulted in the outright starvation of one million people and the emigration of two million (Fry and Goodwin 1997)!

This is a good place to mention that most of the nutrition in potatoes is in the skin. So, buy the smallest ones you can find and scrub them clean before cooking. Why the smallest? The surface area of a ball-shaped object is a function of its radius *squared* while the volume is a function of its radius *cubed*, so the smaller the potato, the more skin relative to volume—a lot more.

The nutritious potato is also a good place to show how Big Food distorts nature's gifts to its commercial ends. The ubiquitous potato chip starts out as that inexpensive, nutritious potato and gets almost its entire nutrition beat out of it as it gets processed for an indefinite shelf life. It is then combined with the terrible trio of added salt, fat, and sugar to make it irresistible (Kessler 2009). On a per-unit weight basis, potato chips' cost can match the most expensive luxury food item you can think of!

Let's now look at what we need to know about eating well from the perspectives of five different stages of nutritional knowledge.

Stage I, Elementary and Middle School

The four-point standard shown below is the crux of a healthy lifestyle:

1. We should eat mainly whole grains, vegetables, unsaturated vegetable oils, fruit, milk and milk products, fish, chicken, eggs, and some meat if we care to. They are real food and the sole content of Mother Nature's pantry.
2. We should not eat unless we are hungry.
3. We should stay away from processed (engineered) foods—in other words sugar, white flour, and white rice.
4. We should get a minimum of fifteen minutes of exercise at least five days each week. A brisk walk or equivalent is all we need. Half an hour is better. A full hour is better yet, but not by much. We are in the area of diminishing returns here.

Exercise in a book on food? Yes! In order to get that food to interact with how we are wired, exercise is critical. A modest level of exercise is all we need (Serdula et al. 1999). Exercising to burn off overindulgence calories is next to impossible, however. It is a lot easier to skip one hamburger in the course of the day than to burn it off by exercise; we would need to walk for an hour and a half!

That's all there is to it. Unless you are a student of physiology, you don't need to know more.

Would you like to know a little more anyway?

Stage II, High School

At this stage we begin to understand, in broad general terms, some of the work of stage IV and V professionals.

Stage III, Undergraduate University Health Sciences Programs

At this stage, the physiology of eating, digestion, absorption and elimination becomes clear. This stage is the training camp for stages IV and V.

Stage IV, Health Professional

At this stage, dietitians, physicians, nurses, midwives, veterinarians, and of course, dentists, apply the investigational findings coming from stage V. At this stage, professionals conduct a lot of good scientific research and clinical trials. The general surgeon, Thomas Cleave, who was the originator of the central tenet of this book (that dental decay is a reliable predictor of obesity, the deadly quartet, and other systemic diseases in later life), was a stage IV professional.

Stage V, Graduate and Postgraduate

Nutrition science is as complex as brain surgery or nuclear physics. At this stage, the best minds with the best training working in the best centers dedicated to the subject toil daily to extract the next nugget of truth. It is here that they understand Mother Nature's inner workings at a molecular and atomic level. Nobel Prize winners in physiology originate here.

In practical terms, that is, as far as eating and lifestyle are concerned, the advanced stages have no advantage over stage I.

It is noteworthy that those who are at stages IV and V, the real experts, universally agree that eating from Mother Nature's pantry is the best possible lifestyle and diet and can prevent all diseases of civilization.

Sustainable Weight Loss

The world does not need yet another diet book, and this is not one. The focal point of this book is to draw attention to the established fact that eating habits that result in dental decay in early life reliably predict the arrival of the diseases of civilization in later life. Dental decay, the first to appear, is the early warning system for any of the others, which, once again, include excess weight and obesity, type 2 diabetes, elevated blood fats, hypertension, and constipation with its consequences—varicose veins, varicocele, hemorrhoids, deep venous thrombosis, and diverticulitis. Researchers are investigating a similar diet link to other ailments including acne, kidney disease, age-related memory decline, and more.

Since concerns with excess weight are a worldwide obsession in all societies that have departed from Mother Nature's pantry, we'll look at that subject more closely. To refocus with emphasis, let me repeat a line from chapter 10 that focuses on excess weight and obesity: "In nature, during periods of food abundance all animals increase the size of their populations, not the size of their bodies."

When living in harmony with our design, we human animals do exactly the same. Today's few remaining hunter–gatherer societies demonstrate that this is the case, as do populations with limited access to engineered food. The Cleave–Yudkin hypothesis has consistently withstood careful scrutiny. Excess weight would be rare if we were not surrounded at every turn by cheap, *engineered*, highly palatable food, concocted to be nearly addictive and pushed by in-your-face marketing pressure.

The only way to lose weight is to burn more calories than we consume. All diets work for that reason and that reason alone. To lose weight, eat less, move more. To maintain the result, the amount of calories you consume (calories in) needs to equal the amount of calories you use (calories out).

Hunger is the number one barrier to weight loss and proper weight maintenance. Mother Nature's pantry only contains ingredients that control hunger.

Counting calories is notoriously difficult. Don't even try. There are better ways of ensuring that calories in equals calories out.

The calories-per-serving (CPS) ratio and/or portion control methods (both described below) are easier than counting calories.

The Calories-Per-Serving (CPS) Ratio
Method for Tracking Calories

If you have the slightest mathematical inclination, you will like the CPS ratio method.

To track CPS, look at the calories in one serving of any food and divide that number by the food's weight in grams or volume in milliliters.

If the quotient is less than 1 (most fruits, vegetables, and low-fat dairy products will be) you can eat any amount. This should be a large portion of *any* diet, especially when weight loss is an objective.

Foods with quotients between 1 and 2 (whole grain bread, brown rice, beans, fish, and fat-free, skinless chicken fall into this category) should make up the rest of any weight-loss diet.

Foods whose quotients are greater than 2 (butter, oil, gravy, ice cream, and nuts, to name a few) should make up small amounts of any weight-loss diet.

Portion Control

Portion control really means calorie control here. There are several methods. The simplest is the plate system: half fill your plate with fruits or vegetables, quarter fill it with lean protein, and quarter fill it with whole grains. Stage IV and V experts recommend that 2:1:1 ratio of carbohydrates to proteins to fats.

A tomato, lettuce, ham, and cheese sandwich can have the same optimal proportions as the plate system. So can any sandwich.

To lose weight, simply reduce your usual portion sizes by about 10 percent until you reach your objective. Greater portion size reduction results in even greater weight loss. However, if the percentage reduction is too great, going down to 1,400 daily calories or less, the risk of micronutrient deficiency increases. Supervision by a physician or registered dietitian is a good idea.

It is well known that activity level is a major determinant of caloric requirements. To lose weight, eat less and move more.

But what about age? With aging comes a reduction of caloric needs. Without an offsetting reduction in caloric consumption, this is the reason why so many people put on one pound of weight for every one year of marriage. It is the aging and not the marriage that causes this gain.

Visit two government-hosted, nutritional Web sites (located at www.mypyramid.gov and www.hc-sc.gc.ca) for portion control information that focuses on calorie control.

Analysis of Popular Weight-Loss Diets

Stage IV and V experts universally agree that one to two pounds a week is the ideal weight-loss rate. Since one pound of fat has 3,500 calories, we need to trim about 500 calories a day to shed excess fat sensibly. Trimming significantly more than that increases our risk of micronutrient deficiency, and the supervision of a physician or registered dietitian is a good idea.

All weight-loss diets ever put together result in initial loss of weight. Not one is based on revolutionary or groundbreaking information, although the most intensively marketed ones assert that they are. Claims that these diets are derived from medical breakthroughs, promises they will provide more than weight loss alone (muscle building without exercise, spot reduction, increased energy, and fat-burning food combinations, to name a few), and contentions that they are *the* magic weight-loss secrets are marketing tactics. No diets, not even the scientifically legitimate ones, are better than the United States and Canadian governments' recommendations for nutrition: My Pyramid (found at www.

89

mypyramid.gov) and Canada's Food Guide (located at www.hc-sc. gc.ca).

When visiting these two excellent sites, keep in mind that governments serve many constituencies, including corporations with deep pockets. Corporations provide millions of jobs, pay millions in taxes, contribute to all conventional political parties, and maintain stables of lobbyists. ConAgra Foods, Florida Crystals, Hershey, Kraft, Krispy Kreme, Mars, Unilever, and others corporations are not entities that any government wants to trifle with. Accordingly, government agencies use weak cautionary language when stronger would be better.

On the other hand, I am free to advise readers to stay away from nutritional crimes—empty-calorie fare, engineered foods, soft drinks, energy drinks, white flour products, heavily advertized snacks, cereals, the terrible trio foods that combine salt, fat, and added sugar, and any other engineered foods that hunters and gatherers would not recognize. Indeed, our grandparents would not recognize them!

My Pyramid allows for "discretionary calories," allowing some room for nutritional crimes (consuming foods with empty calories and zero nutritional value). Why allow them into our lives at all? The Canadian guidelines encourage visitors to "limit" foods and beverages high in calories, fat, sugar, or salt (sodium). Why "limit" instead of "avoid"? I can easily suggest that we avoid them completely. This book has no corporate sponsors.

Significantly, scientific studies show that, when it comes to weight loss, the macronutrient balance of a diet is irrelevant. In other words, the labels "low carb," "high carb," "low fat," "high fat," "low protein," "high protein" don't matter.

To check the soundness of any diet that might interest you, simply make sure that it meets the four healthy lifestyle points noted above in "Stage I, Elementary and Middle School." For a science-based outline of fifty most popular diets, WebMD, located at www. webmd.com, is an excellent source. Every one of the diets reviewed is effective in the short term.

To check requirements for long-term, successful weight-loss maintenance, review the findings of the National Weight Control Registry (www.nwcr.ws). Launched by stage V experts nearly two decades ago, the registry follows over five thousand people who have lost thirty pounds or more and kept it off for at least one year. In fact, for registry participants, the average weight loss is seventy pounds, and the average period of weight loss maintenance is six years! There are no common elements among weight-loss diets used—none at all. Again, all weight-loss diets work. However, for weight-loss maintenance, there are four indispensable, ever-present requirements:

1. Regular movement (exercise)
2. Regular weighing
3. Regular breakfast
4. No more than 25 percent dietary fat

As to movement (exercise), registry participants exercise (mainly walking) an hour a day on average. Many don't necessarily love it. Like brushing teeth or washing dishes, it is simply a part of their lives.

Regularly weighing yourself provides the early warning system for any backsliding. A weight check that shows a gain signals when it's time to start corrective action while it is relatively easy to do so.

Experts have long seen the importance of breakfast in appetite control, weight control, and dietary quality. Breakfast is currently attracting increasing interest among stage IV and V experts within the scientific community.

Finally, limiting fats to 25 percent of your caloric intake is in line with experts' advice (that you should eat carbs, proteins, and fats, according to a 2:1:1 ratio respectively).

Diet Categories

Any of the hundreds of diets out there fall into one of five categories. There is some overlap, and several of the diets fall into more than one category.

Category 1. Mother Nature's Lifestyle Diets

We know that Mother Nature's pantry only offers whole grains, vegetables, unsaturated vegetable oils, fruit, milk and milk products, fish, chicken, eggs, and some meat on its shelves. There are no refined carbohydrates (sugar, white flour, and white rice).

These diets and lifestyles respect our ancient and genetically determined biology. They pay attention to the Stone Age nutritional and activity requirements that we are wired for. They are our ancestral diets of millions of years ago and are in harmony with our design. Here is a brief review of several popular ones.

Best Life Diet
Experts hold this diet in high regard; it promotes Mother Nature's pantry. Put together by exercise physiologist Bob Greene, this diet is based on solid science, is easy to follow, and promotes the healthy lifestyle *Your Mouth, Your Health: Stop and Reverse Aging* supports.

Biggest Loser Diet
Backed by a popular TV show, this diet promotes Mother Nature's pantry and gets high marks from experts. It is centered on a 4-3-2-1 pyramid made up of four servings of fruits and vegetables, three of lean protein, two of whole grains, and one "extra." This is a slight variation on the Portion Control method described above and embodies the same principles.

Dr. Phil's Ultimate Weight Solution
We know that the mathematical answer to sustainable weight loss is elementary. However, the obsession with diets and the huge industry it has spawned shows that there is a good deal more to it than simple calorie-counting arithmetic. Enter the psychology of overeating. In its marketing activities, Big Food effectively uses its deep understanding of emotions and eating to put more calories into us. The psychology of overeating is a major focus of Big Food marketing.

Phil McGraw, PhD, shows how to combine the control of emotional and impulsive overeating with exercise into a lifestyle.

The diet gets high marks for advocating food from Mother Nature's panty and opposing refined carbohydrates (added sugar and white flour).

The downside of Dr. Phil's outstanding approach to healthy living is that it recommends that we put a lot of labor and effort into food preparation. No one has shown the benefits of that approach, whereas the time cost is clear.

Glycemic Index Diet (Low Glycemic Diet)
Searching for foods best suited for diabetics, Dr. David Jenkins and University of Toronto colleagues developed the glycemic index (GI) in 1980–1981. It is still being fine-tuned. Based on solid science, the GI distinguishes between carbohydrates that are digested slowly (those in Mother Nature's pantry), those that are digested quickly (refined carbohydrates), and those that lie in between. Using either glucose or white bread as reference points, the GI assigns relative values to carbohydrates and makes sensible selection possible.

The GI is foundational to several popular diets such as *South Beach* and *The Zone* and many others.

Selecting carbohydrates with low GIs, combined with lean protein, healthy fats, and regular physical activity might well help those who haven't succeeded on other diets.

Jenny Craig Weight Loss Program
The program originated in Australia over thirty years ago. Its three-level dietary and psychological program is in keeping with eating sensibly from Mother Nature's pantry and being active.

There is a 24/7 telephone support line available to clients in either of its two programs. One is based on participating in one of over 650 Jenny Craig centers, and the other is an at-home program supported by mail or phone.

Central to the program are prepackaged, frozen meals based on sound dietary principles. Visit the company's Web site (www. jennycraig.com) for a detailed introduction.

Medifast Diet Plan

Launched nearly three decades ago, this $300-a-month meal replacement program is supervised and available through the company's Web site (www.medifast1.com). It promotes eating from Mother Nature's pantry and is a simple approach, first to weight loss and then to healthy living. Stage IV and V experts regard this program highly.

Mayo Clinic Diet

The *real* Mayo Clinic Diet is an outstanding guide to adopting a healthy lifestyle. Don't confuse it with the phony "Mayo Clinic Diet" described below under the "Bizarre Diets" heading. The Mayo Clinic Web site, located at www.mayoclinic.com, offers diet details, in addition to other sound, science-based health recommendations. Getting the free e-mail newsletter is a worthwhile way for the layperson to keep abreast of health issues.

The *real* Mayo Clinic Diet promotes the four following points:

1. The Mayo Clinic Healthy Weight Pyramid
2. Physical activity
3. Realistic goals
4. Ongoing motivation.

Mediterranean Diet

Looking into the relationship between coronary heart disease and saturated fats consumption nearly twenty-five years ago, the Seven Countries Study discovered that the Greek island, Crete, had the lowest rate of heart disease among these countries (Keys et al. 1986). Numerous studies looking into what became known as the Mediterranean Diet followed. The evidence is clear in regards to this diet, which is not much different from the way hunter–gatherer societies ate. It not only results in highest average life expectancy but also prevents and even reverses heart disease. It is the best way to eat to prevent all the diseases of civilization, each of which starts as dental decay, unless high-tech dentistry prevents it.

The Mediterranean Diet consists of:

1. Unrefined carbohydrates (whole grain bread, pasta, and brown rice); fruit and vegetables; and beans and nuts daily
2. Fish, poultry, and eggs four to five times weekly
3. Red meat four to five times monthly

The main added fat is olive oil and, good news, this diet encourages two glasses of wine daily with meals, as well as being physically active.

Nutrition for Dummies
The diet-related sections of this "For Dummies" book are as sound as the other aspects of nutrition it deals with. Recommendations are supported by mainstream science references, and the index is comprehensive. Like every "For Dummies" book, the subtitle, "A Reference for the Rest of Us!" portrays the book's nonthreatening approach to a complex subject. The dieting recommendations squarely meet the four healthy lifestyle points noted above in "Stage I, Elementary and Middle School."

NutriSystem Diet
In keeping with ongoing changes in the world of science, this forty-year-old program is now solidly in the low glycemic index camp. It provides healthy, prepackaged, microwaveable meals and is as convenient as it gets.

The diet meets our four-point healthy lifestyle standard, provides solid textbook and newsletter advice, as well as telephone counseling. Whether dieters can sustain results on their own once they quit NutriSystem is questionable.

Okinawa Diet
People from Okinawa claim the longest life expectancy in the world, although Mediterranean diet-eating residents of Crete make the same claim. These claims are, in part, due to the diets on these islands.

Okinawans' diets are lower in calories than Japanese diets—leaving the table while still slightly hungry is a cultural practice.

The diet relies heavily on sweet potatoes and other vegetables and includes small amounts of fat-free pork and of fish.

The commercialized version monitors the caloric density of foods, much like the CPS ratio described at the beginning of this chapter.

Slim-Fast Weight Loss Plan

The company behind this diet offers a highly ordered plan of activity, sensible eating, portion control, and support. Slim-Fast offers a line of meal-replacement products that can take the thinking out of eating properly. The program is backed by sound research and involves eating six small meals every day.

The company's comprehensive Web site (www.slim-fast.com) offers counseling, support, and products for sale.

Weight Watchers Diet

Solidly science-based, this fifty-year-old guide to the healthy lifestyle is held in high regards among stage IV and V experts. Weight Watchers changes constantly to stay in line with the latest nutritional scientific findings and addresses lifestyle as a whole. The cornerstones of this balanced and comprehensive approach deal with smarter eating, more movement, support, and smarter habits.

Weil's Diet (Dr. Andrew)

Stage IV and V experts give this diet high marks for standing on sound, accepted nutritional principles in a common-sense way. It combines Eastern lifestyle approaches with Western ones and is especially useful for lactose-intolerant people. This is almost a vegetarian diet, but it includes small amounts of animal products. For a closer look, visit www.drweil.com.

You: On a Diet: The Owner's Manual for Waist Management

This science-based approach to eating and lifestyle incorporates the four points at the beginning of this chapter (eat from Mother Nature's pantry, don't eat unless you are hungry, don't eat processed [engineered] foods like sugar, white flour, and white rice, and get some exercise).

Instead of regularly weighing yourself, which almost all successful dieters do, this book stresses monitoring your waist size. The substitution is absolutely acceptable. The key is in the monitoring.

Category 2. High-Protein Diets

Collectively these diets do not have much respect among stage IV and V experts. High-protein diets claim that the overweight eat too many carbohydrates, whereas we know that the overweight simply eat too much (Foster et al. 2003).

Atkins Diet
This is a well-known example of a high-protein diet. It was a huge commercial success, right up to the death of Dr. Robert Atkins, its founder and driving force. When he died after a fall at age seventy-two, he was obese and had heart disease.

Body for Life Diet
This is another high-protein diet with a strong emphasis on exercise. Stage IV and V experts feel that most people would find the recommended workouts difficult to stick with.

Category 3. Vegetarian and Vegan Lifestyle Diets

Vegetarians who eat eggs and milk products tend to have higher than average levels of health. However, much of that comes from their greater than average health awareness and accompanying lifestyle. Many vegetarian and all vegan (no egg or milk products allowed) diets go counter to the conventional nutritional wisdom, which this book is founded on. Nevertheless, since most North Americans don't eat enough plant foods, stage IV and V professionals approve of vegetarian diets if tempered by supplementation. Calcium, iodine, iron, protein, riboflavin, vitamin D, and zinc are especially difficult to get on an undisciplined vegetarian diet, and bioavailable vitamin B_{12} and omega-3 fatty acids are only available from animal products.

The anthropologic record shows that we are omnivores. To blend into our environment in the manner for which we are wired requires us to include animal products in our diets (Blumenschine et al. 1987).

A trendy, new way of eating, the *Raw Food Diet,* is another variation of vegetarianism. Also called raw foodism or rawism, allowing for the caveats described here, this diet largely meets with the approval of stage IV and V experts. Raw foodists spend a lot of time in the kitchen peeling, chopping, blending, dehydrating, and handling their basic ingredients in ways that have little solid science to support their claims. Rawism preparation methods are rituals with their own unique appeal for some.

Category 4. Hard-to-Categorize Diets

These interesting but indefinable diets are included for the sake of completeness.

Eat This, Not That
Strictly speaking, this is not a diet book but a practical guide for making sensible selections in fast food restaurants where, much of the time, commercial considerations are totally misaligned with nutritional ones. "Eat This" foods are printed on one side of the page and "Not That" foods on the other. With regular use, the book's content will become an internalized response when looking over fast food restaurant menus.

French Women Don't Get Fat
The accurate title for this book might be *French Women Didn't Get Fat.* As fast food, with the related increase in refined carbohydrates, begins to replace traditional French dining styles, the obesity rate in France is on the rise.

French women didn't get fat partly because they smoked and still do, so they curb their appetites. But the traditional French lifestyle did include the enjoyment of small amounts of high quality food and wine coupled with daily walking. No food was off limits, but large portions were—not a bad way to go through life. The information in *French Women Don't Get Fat: The Secret of Eating for*

Pleasure can be adjusted to meet *Your Mouth, Your Health* tenets and is worth looking into.

Pritikin Principle

Limited to 10 percent of calories from fat—one of the lowest limits anywhere—this diet is mainly based on vegetables, grains, and fruits. Exercise is accorded proper respect, and stress-reduction is a part of the program.

Fat inhibits stomach emptying more than any of the other macronutrients, and so it staves off hunger longer. The extremely low fat content of the Pritikin diet virtually guarantees prolonged feelings of hunger, the number one enemy of any sustained dietary program. Further, there is a risk of missing out on fat-soluble vitamins (A, D, E, and K). These are two important reasons why stage IV and V experts recommend a 2:1:1 carbohydrates-protein-fats ratio.

The Pritikin Longevity Center and Spa in Miami (located online at www.pritikin.com) has been in operation for decades and is aimed at people with thick middles and thick wallets. Once they leave that protected environment, sticking with the diet is unrealistic.

For folk of average income, a lot of printed material is available.

The Zone Diet

Barry Sears, PhD, spent fifteen years as a stage V scientist in nutrition research. His scientific credentials are above reproach. However, he and his co-author, Bill Lawren, have turned their backs on respected nutrition science and state that much of it is "dead wrong." For that reason alone, I cannot place their recommendations on the "Mother Nature's Lifestyle Diets" list.

The Zone Diet is one of many founded on Jenkins's Glycemic Index principles, with unique theories added in. The theories are supported by "scientific" rhetoric but not by scientific documentation.

Category 5. Bizarre Diets

Selling to the ingenuous, the ingenious have created an industry out of many of the diets listed below. Diets in this category are dangerous in the long run, even though they are effective initially. You might want to go on one to kick-start a weight-loss program, with the objective of changing to one of Mother Nature's Lifestyle Diets when you reach your weight objective. Starting out and staying on any of Mother Nature's Lifestyle Diets is better.

Cabbage Soup Diet
Some hospitals recommend this broth-based vegetable soup for patients who need to drop a few pounds quickly to make elective surgery safer. There is no controversy among experts about the fact that this diet is a prescription for disaster in the long term.

Cheater's Diet
Authored by Paul Rivas, MD, this is the Mediterranean diet with regular exercise allowing for "cheating" on weekends—36 hours for each 168-hour week. Permitted cheat foods are both energy dense and nutrient dense, with no empty calories permitted. Examples are bread, pizza, chocolate, peanut butter, ice cream, meat, nuts, and cheese.

Our caveman body is designed to conserve energy during periods of food shortages so it slows down our metabolic rate, our fuel-burning speed if you like, during extreme low-calorie diets. Once off a diet, our caveman body ensures that we eat a lot to prepare for the next food shortage. That is why the yo-yo effect is so common among dieters. Rivas claims that the cheating prevents the yo-yo effect but provides no references or research to support these claims.

Further, the diet recommends some peculiar dietary supplements. For a review of the science behind supplementation, see chapter 6, "Vitamins and Minerals: Need Turned to Hoax."

Cookie Diet
This diet replaces breakfast, lunch, and snacks with about 500 calories worth of cookies, said to suppress hunger by the nature of

their composition. Dieters are allowed dinner ranging from 300 to 1,000 calories. Fruit is off limits, and exercise is not a part of the program. Accordingly, the diet fails to meet the four-point standard of a healthy lifestyle, even though following it will result in weight loss.

Eat Right for Your Blood Type Diet

In this diet, people's blood type (A, B, AB, or O) determines what foods they should or should not eat. The dietary recommendations are fine, but the reasoning behind them is unsupported by published, peer-reviewed science. From the perspectives of stages III, IV and V, this is amusing stuff.

Fruit Flush Diet

Eating fruit every two hours is central to the Fruit Flush, three-day detox diet. Coupled with protein shakes, this diet claims to relieve the body of the "digestive burden" of eating from other food groups, as well as to "detox" the body or flush out wastes.

Based on shaky science, this diet is blind to our body's superb design to handle a wide range of foods, as well as to "detox" itself via the colon, kidneys, lungs, liver, and skin.

Following this diet will result in rapid initial weight loss, about half of it being water. It is not a good lifestyle way of eating.

The 100-Mile Diet: A Year of Local Eating

Devoid of nutritional science, supported by celebs without a science background, the feel-good local food or "locavore" movement is sweeping the land. Eating food produced within a one hundred–mile radius of where we live is supposed to reduce the carbon footprint of long-distance food transportation. The claim fails to stand up to even minimal fact-checking. Container transport of thousands of cases of strawberries over thousands of miles by truck, rail, and ship leaves a much smaller carbon footprint per strawberry than transporting ten cases over ten miles by a farmer's pickup truck, however romantic the latter may be.

The hundred-mile way of eating gives no nutritional or dietary advice, and adherents deprive themselves of many outstanding foods from Mother Nature's pantry that simply cannot be produced locally. This is one advantage we have over hunter-gatherer societies, whose diets aligned with the way we are designed.

Supporting local farmers and eating fresher and possibly better-tasting food can be a reason to be a "locavore." Being a flexivore is better. Support local farmers, but don't shortchange yourself on foods they are geographically and climatologically unable to grow.

Macrobiotic Diet

Even though the word *macrobiotic* comes from Greek, meaning "great life," the origin of this diet (or more correctly, this way of life) is Japanese. It combines a Western vegetarian diet with Zen mysticism and balances foods described as having "yin" and "yang" qualities.

The original version required adherents to restrict their diets increasingly as they progressed along the path toward enlightenment, until they got to a point at which they could only eat brown rice and water! Today, those who follow the modified macrobiotic way of life are locavores who follow the equivalent of the Mediterranean diet using traditionally prepared ingredients. Not surprisingly, given its Japanese source, this diet emphasizes soy products.

Completely bereft of a science-based foundation, some variations of this diet are an example of doing the right thing for the wrong reasons.

Martha's Vineyard Diet Detox: Lose 21 Pounds in 21 Days

The word "detox" alone in the name of this diet should raise a red flag. So should its recommendations for weekly coffee enemas, a "passive aerobic exerciser," an annual twenty-one-day detox, a quarterly seven-day cleanup, and a weekly two-day detox. This quirky plan based on shaky science would be dangerous in the long run. Check it out for amusement only.

The "Mayo Clinic" Diet

Riding on the fame and reputation of the respected Minnesota Mayo Clinic, the "Mayo Clinic" Diet is a fake name with no connection to the authentic Mayo Clinic. It has been around for eighty years or more and attributes miraculous fat-burning powers to grapefruit. It claims wonders and focuses on avoiding complex carbohydrates, the very food from Mother Nature's pantry we need in order to avoid the diseases of civilization. This phony "Mayo Clinic" Diet is a prescription for dietary disaster and is best read for amusement.

Morning Banana Diet

Promoted as the easiest and fastest way to lose weight, this diet attributes magic fat-burning properties to bananas. We know that neither bananas nor any other foods burn fat. This false claim, coupled with the fact that it recommends no exercise, demonstrates that this diet rests on rickety science.

New Beverly Hills Diet

Enthusiastic but innocent, Judy Mazel, the author of this diet, had no formal training in nutrition when she wrote her book. A huge commercial success with celebrity endorsements, this diet is another example of the victory of marketing over science. It theorizes that exercise is irrelevant, calories don't count, and combining foods correctly is the ideal way to lose weight. Stage IV and V experts universally agree that this diet is a contender for the top spot among quirky fad diets.

Organic Food Diets

Today's crop enhancers (formerly called agricultural chemicals), together with plant and animal breeding and irrigation improvement, are enormous advances and the logical extensions of what farmers have done since farming began. Culminating in the Green Revolution in the middle of the twentieth century, modern farming is saving millions from hunger, malnutrition, and starvation.

Much of "organic food" production is simply a step backward to the idyllic but ineffective methods that preceded the Green Revolution. Organic food has a significant marketing advantage when aimed at certain niche groups, but it has no nutritional advantage over any other real food.

Paleolithic (Old Stone Age) Diet

This is the Mediterranean Diet minus grains, legumes, and dairy products. It consists of fruits, vegetables, root vegetables, eggs, nuts, lean meat, and fish, and it assumes that this is how hominins ate before the agricultural revolution beginning about ten thousand years ago. In two small, high quality scientific studies, the Paleolithic Diet did get better results in heart disease and type 2 diabetic patients than the Mediterranean Diet or a diet specifically designed for diabetics.

While the essential evolutionary logic of the Paleolithic Diet is appealing, stage IV and V experts put it on their fad diet list, questioning its accuracy.

Grains, a no-no on this diet, have a key role in the agricultural revolution, and 96 percent of today's annual two billion tons goes into human food and animal feed. (About 4 percent is used for fuel.) The Paleolithic Diet on a global scale is simply not possible.

In Conclusion

You can safely rely on the four-point standards listed in "Stage I, Elementary and Middle School" for the best possible lifestyle and diet to prevent and even reverse any one of the diseases of civilization. Since the topic of diets is common at social gatherings, you can use this book as a reference source for science-based positions on nutrition. Armed with that information, balance your knowledge of science with an understanding of the humanities and go about your business of living your life to the fullest.

Conclusion:
For Policymakers:
A Proven Results System

We North Americans are among the most overfed and malnourished societies in history. The resulting diseases are the subject of this book. Their cost in diminished quality of life is appalling. Their economic cost is astronomic. Their rate of increase is frightening.

What would it take for North Americans to be healthier? It is not a mystery (Temple and Burkitt 1993). A lot of factors contribute to the problems of North American malnutrition, but two major ones are aggressive marketing of unhealthy food and decreased activity.

Unhealthy food today is what tobacco was a generation ago. History shows that cigarette price increases due to taxes reduce cigarette sales and consumption (American Cancer Society 2000). A reduction in cigarette sales and consumption saves lives (Smith and Glynn 2000). That is, history shows that the most effective cure for lung cancer didn't come from medical research but from government policy (Polednak 2008). Stated another way, the biggest breakthrough in health care in the last generation was not a new cancer treatment, the CT scan, the MRI, a new drug, or another hospital wing, but increased taxation on cigarettes.

Similarly, the best cure for North America's malnutrition will not be a medical approach but the right mix of taxes and subsidies to promote healthier lifestyles.

Almost two hundred years ago, the U.S. Supreme Court Chief Justice John Marshall stated that the power to tax is the power to destroy. It was ever thus. Conversely, the power to subsidize is the power to develop. Using that basic principle, policymakers can promote healthier lifestyles by tearing down the forces promoting our malnutrition and inactivity and supporting the forces that encourage healthy lifestyles. Judiciously and incrementally taxing the former and using the revenue gained to subsidize the latter will get positive results, as the tobacco story proves. The right balance of taxes and subsidies will encourage consumers to buy healthier foods and become more active. Introducing the needed changes gradually would not be disruptive. All concerned would be winners.

We know the lifestyle requirements for health and longevity. It is time we implemented them into our policies.

Policymakers could create an advisory council to consult with existing agriculture, food, and biotechnology industries and associations in order to bring about the needed changes.

Consumer education could start as early as the first grade of school. After a period of several years of consumer education, governments could slowly decrease health care coverage for conditions proven to be brought on by an unhealthy lifestyle.

Additional to increased tax revenue, the resulting savings on health care could subsidize food groups and behaviors known to promote health.

With no additional cost to taxpayers, policymakers could implement tactics that, over time, would move North Americans from being among the most overfed, malnourished societies in history to being among the healthiest.

References

Introduction: Most Chronic Disease is a Choice

Allam, Adel H., Randall C. Thompson, L. Samuel Wann, Michael I. Miyamoto, and Gregory S. Thomas. 2009. Computed tomographic assessment of atherosclerosis in ancient Egyptian mummies. *JAMA: The Journal of the American Medical Association* 302(19) (November 18): 2091– 94. doi: 10.1001/jama.2009.1641.

Cleave, Thomas. 1974. *The Saccharine Disease: The Master Disease of Our Time.* Bristol: John Wright and Sons Limited.

Cordain, Loren, S. Boyd Eaton, Anthony Sebastian, Neil Mann, Staffan Lindeberg, Bruce A. Watkins, James H. O'Keefe, and Janette Brand-Miller. 2005. Origins and evolution of the Western diet: Health implications for the 21st century. *The American Journal of Clinical Nutrition* 81(2) (February): 341– 54.

Eaton, S. B. 2000. Paleolithic vs. modern diets—Selected pathophysiological implications. *European Journal of Nutrition* 39(2) (April): 67–70.

Hujoel, P. 2009. Dietary carbohydrates and dental-systemic diseases. *Journal of Dental Research* 88(6) (June): 490–502. doi: 10.1177/0022034509337700.

Johnson, Rachel K., Lawrence J. Appel, Michael Brands, Barbara V. Howard, Michael Lefevre, Robert H. Lustig, Frank Sacks, Lyn M. Steffen, and Judith Wylie-Rosett. 2009. Dietary sugars intake and cardiovascular health: A scientific statement from the American Heart Association.

Circulation 120(11) (September 15): 1011– 20. doi: 10.1161/ CIRCULATIONAHA.109.192627.

Richards, Michael P. 2002. A brief review of the archaeological evidence for Palaeolithic and Neolithic subsistence. *European Journal of Clinical Nutrition* 56(12) (December): 1270–78. doi: 10.1038/sj.ejcn.1601646.

Temple, N. J. and D. P. Burkitt. 1993. Towards a new system of health: The challenge of Western disease. *Journal of Community Health* 18(1) (February): 37– 47.

CHAPTER 1.
OUR BODIES: HOW WE (AND EVERYTHING ELSE) ARE BUILT

Bobbio, A. 1973. [Maya, the first authentic alloplastic, endosseous dental implant. A refinement of a priority]. *Revista Da Associação Paulista De Cirurgiões Dentistas* 27(1) (February): 27–36.

Davies, W. Paul. 2003. An historical perspective from the Green Revolution to the gene revolution. *Nutrition Reviews* 61(6) (June): S124–34.

Hirst, K. Krist. 2010. Hominin. *About.com.* http://archaeology. about.com/od/hterms/g/hominin.htm.

Magkos, Faidon, Fotini Arvaniti, and Antonis Zampelas. 2003. Organic food: Nutritious food or food for thought? A review of the evidence. *International Journal of Food Sciences and Nutrition* 54(5) (September): 357–71. doi: 10.1080/09637480120092071.

Richards, Michael P. 2002. A brief review of the archaeological evidence for Palaeolithic and Neolithic subsistence. *European Journal of Clinical Nutrition* 56(12) (December): 1270–78. doi: 10.1038/sj.ejcn.1601646.

Strathern, Paul. 2001. *Mendeleyev's Dream: The Quest for the Elements.* New York: St. Martins Press.

Temple, N. J. and D. P. Burkitt. 1993. Towards a new system of health: The challenge of Western disease. *Journal of Community Health* 18(1) (February): 37–47.

CHAPTER 2.
CARBOHYDRATES: THE MISUNDERSTOOD ENERGY

Gunnarsdottir, Ingibjorg, Annette Due, Leila Karhunen, and Marika Lyly. 2009. [Can health claims made on food be scientifically substantiated? Review on satiety and weight management]. *Læknabladid* 95(3) (March): 195–200.

Hernot, David, Thomas Boileau, Laura Bauer, Kelly Swanson, and George Fahey. 2008. In Vitro Digestion Characteristics of Unprocessed and Processed Whole Grains and Their Components. *Journal of Agricultural and Food Chemistry* (November 5).

Hujoel, P. 2009. Dietary carbohydrates and dental-systemic diseases. *Journal of Dental Research* 88(6) (June): 490–502. doi: 10.1177/0022034509337700.

Kopp, Wolfgang. 2003. High-insulinogenic nutrition—An etiologic factor for obesity and the metabolic syndrome? *Metabolism: Clinical and Experimental* 52(7) (July): 840–44.

———. 2005. Pathogenesis and etiology of essential hypertension: Role of dietary carbohydrate. *Medical Hypotheses* 64(4): 782–87. doi: 10.1016/j.mehy.2004.10.009.

———. 2006. The atherogenic potential of dietary carbohydrate. *Preventive Medicine* 42(5) (May): 336–42. doi: 10.1016/j.ypmed.2006.02.003.

Malik, Vasanti S., Matthias B. Schulze, and Frank B. Hu. 2006. Intake of sugar-sweetened beverages and weight gain: A systematic review. *The American Journal of Clinical Nutrition* 84(2) (August): 274–88.

Sarter, Barbara, T. Colin Campbell, and Joel Fuhrman. 2008. Effect of a high nutrient density diet on long-term weight loss: A retrospective chart review. *Alternative Therapies in Health and Medicine* 14(3) (June): 48–53.

CHAPTER 3.
PROTEINS: LIFE'S BLUEPRINT

Barbour, Michele E., R. Peter Shellis, David M. Parker, Geoff C. Allen, and Martin Addy. 2008. Inhibition of hydroxyapatite dissolution by whole casein: The effects of pH, protein concentration, calcium, and ionic strength. *European Journal of Oral Sciences* 116(5) (October): 473–78. doi: 10.1111/j.1600-0722.2008.00565.x.

Craig, Winston J. and Ann Reed Mangels. 2009. Position of the American Dietetic Association: Vegetarian diets. *Journal of the American Dietetic Association* 109(7) (July): 1266–82.

Ferrazzano, G. F., T. Cantile, M. Quarto, A. Ingenito, L. Chianese, and F. Addeo. 2008. Protective effect of yogurt extract on dental enamel demineralization in vitro. *Australian Dental Journal* 53(4) (December): 314–19. doi: 10.1111/j.1834-7819.2008.00072.x.

Haimel, Matthias, Karin Pröll, and Michael Rebhan. 2009. ProteinArchitect: Protein evolution above the sequence level. *PloS One* 4(7): e6176. doi: 10.1371/journal.pone.0006176.

Sire, Jean-Yves, Tiphaine Davit-Béal, Sidney Delgado, and Xun Gu. 2007. The origin and evolution of enamel mineralization genes. *Cells, Tissues, Organs* 186(1): 25–48. doi: 10.1159/000102679.

CHAPTER 4.
FATS: LOVE THEM, YOU CAN'T LEAVE THEM

Ascherio, A., E. B. Rimm, E. L. Giovannucci, D. Spiegelman, M. Stampfer, and W. C. Willett. 1996. Dietary fat and risk of coronary heart disease in men: Cohort follow up study in the United States. *BMJ (Clinical Research Ed.)* 313(7,049) (July 13): 84–90.

Ascherio, A. and W. C. Willett. 1997. Health effects of trans fatty acids. *American Journal of Clinical Nutrition* 66(4) (October 1): 1006S–1010.

Eckel, Robert H., Penny Kris-Etherton, Alice H. Lichtenstein, Judith Wylie-Rosett, Allison Groom, Kimberly F. Stitzel, and Shirley Yin-Piazza. 2009. Americans' awareness, knowledge, and behaviors regarding fats: 2006–2007. *Journal of the American Dietetic Association* 109(2) (February): 288–96. doi: 10.1016/j.jada.2008.10.048.

Government of Canada, Health Canada.2008. An assessment of continuing care requirements in first nations and Inuit communities: Review of literature and national health data sources. *Health Canada*: n.d. 5. http://www.hc-sc.gc.ca/fniah-spnia/pubs/services/_home-domicile/2008_assess-eval-exam/02-research-recher-env-eng.php.

Mensink, R. P., and M. B. Katan. 1990. Effect of dietary trans fatty acids on high-density and low-density lipoprotein cholesterol levels in healthy subjects. *The New England Journal of Medicine* 323(7) (August 16): 439–45.

Motoyama, Kenneth R., J. David Curb, Takashi Kadowaki, Aiman El-Saed, Robert D. Abbott, Tomonori Okamura, Robert W. Evans, et al. 2009. Association of serum n-6 and n-3 polyunsaturated fatty acids with lipids in 3 populations of middle-aged men. *The American Journal of Clinical Nutrition* 90(1) (July): 49–55. doi: 10.3945/ajcn.2008.26761.

Zevenbergen, H., A. de Bree, M. Zeelenberg, K. Laitinen, G. van Duijn, and E. Flöter. 2009. Foods with a high fat quality are essential for healthy diets. *Annals of Nutrition & Metabolism* 54(Suppl 1): 15–24. doi: 10.1159/000220823.

CHAPTER 5.
WATER: NEED TURNED TO MARKETING TRIUMPH

Bray, G. A. 2008. Fructose: Should we worry? *International Journal of Obesity (2005)* 32(Suppl 7) (December): S127–31. doi: 10.1038/ijo.2008.248.

Centers for Disease Control and Prevention. 1999. Ten great public health achievements—United States, 1900–1999. *MMWR. Morbidity and Mortality Weekly Report* 48(12) (April 2): 241–43.

Doria, Miguel F. 2006. Bottled water versus tap water: Understanding consumers' preferences. *Journal of Water and Health* 4(2) (June): 271–76.

Fry, Iris. 2006. The origins of research into the origins of life. *Endeavour* 30(1) (March): 24–28. doi: 10.1016/j.endeavour.2005.12.002.

Gualberto, F. A. S. and L. Heller. 2006. Endemic Cryptosporidium infection and drinking water source: A systematic review and meta-analyses. *Water Science and Technology: A Journal of the International Association on Water Pollution Research* 54(3): 231–38.

Gyntelberg, Finn, Hans Ole Hein, and Poul Suadicani. 2009. Sugar in coffee or tea and risk of obesity: A neglected issue. *International Journal of Food Sciences and Nutrition* 60 (Suppl 3): 56–64.

Kenney, W. L. and P. Chiu. 2001. Influence of age on thirst and fluid intake. *Medicine and Science in Sports and Exercise* 33(9) (September): 1524–32.

Knoops, Kim T. B., C. P. Lisette, G. M. de Groot, Daan Kromhout, Anne-Elisabeth Perrin, Olga Moreiras-Varela, Alessandro Menotti, and Wija A. van Staveren. 2004. Mediterranean diet, lifestyle factors, and 10-year mortality in elderly European men and women: The HALE project. *JAMA: The Journal of the American Medical Association* 292(12) (September 22): 1433–1439. doi: 10.1001/jama.292.12.1433.

Thelin, W. R., M. T. Brennan, P. B. Lockhart, M. L. Singh, P. C. Fox, A. S. Papas, and R. C. Boucher. 2008. The oral mucosa as a therapeutic target for xerostomia. *Oral Diseases* 14(8) (November): 683–89. doi: 10.1111/j.1601-0825.2008.01486.x.

Wolf, A., G. A. Bray, and B. M. Popkin. 2008. A short history of beverages and how our body treats them. *Obesity Reviews: An Official Journal of the International Association for the Study of Obesity* 9, no. 2 (March): 151-164. doi:10.1111/j.1467-789X.2007.00389.x.

CHAPTER 6.
VITAMINS AND MINERALS: NEED TURNED TO HOAX

Bartholomew, M. 2002. James Lind's treatise of the scurvy (1753). *Postgraduate Medical Journal* 78(925) (November): 695–96.

Bjelakovic, G., A. Nagorni, D. Nikolova, R. G. Simonetti, M. Bjelakovic, and C. Gluud. 2006. Meta-analysis: Antioxidant supplements for primary and secondary prevention of colorectal adenoma. *Alimentary Pharmacology & Therapeutics* 24(2) (July 15): 281–91. doi: 10.1111/j.1365-2036.2006.02970.x.

Bjelakovic, G., D. Nikolova, R. G. Simonetti, and C. Gluud. 2008. Systematic review and meta-analysis: Primary and secondary prevention of gastrointestinal cancers with antioxidant supplements. *Alimentary Pharmacology & Therapeutics* (June 30). doi: 10.1111/j.1365-2036.2008.03785.x. http://www.ncbi.nlm.nih.gov/pubmed/18616690.

Blencowe, Hannah, Simon Cousens, Bernadette Modell, and Joy Lawn. 2010. Folic acid to reduce neonatal mortality from neural tube disorders. *International Journal of Epidemiology* 39(Suppl 1) (April): i110–21. doi: 10.1093/ije/dyq028.

Briefel, Ronette, Charlotte Hanson, Mary Kay Fox, Timothy Novak, and Paula Ziegler. 2006. Feeding Infants and Toddlers Study: Do vitamin and mineral supplements contribute to nutrient adequacy or excess among US infants and toddlers? *Journal of the American Dietetic Association* 106(1) (January): S52–65. doi: 10.1016/j.jada.2005.09.041.

Brown, H. K. and M. Poplove. 1965. Brantford-Sarnia-Stratford fluoridation caries study: Final survey, 1963. *Journal of the Canadian Dental Association* 31 (August): 505–11.

Centers for Disease Control and Prevention. 1999. Ten great public health achievements—United States, 1900–1999. *MMWR. Morbidity and Mortality Weekly Report* 48(12): 241–43.

Douglas, R. M., H. Hemilä, E. Chalker, and B. Treacy. 2007. Vitamin C for preventing and treating the common cold. *Cochrane Database of Systematic Reviews (Online)* 3: CD000980. doi: 10.1002/14651858.CD000980.pub3.

Eaton, S. B., and S. B. Eaton III. 2000. Paleolithic vs. modern diets—Selected pathophysiological implications. *European Journal of Nutrition* 39(2) (April): 67–70.

Frassetto, L., R. C. Morris, D. E. Sellmeyer, K. Todd, and A. Sebastian. 2001. Diet, evolution and aging—The pathophysiologic effects of the post-agricultural inversion of the potassium-to-sodium and base-to-chloride ratios in the human diet. *European Journal of Nutrition* 40(5) (October): 200–213.

Gennari, C. 2001. Calcium and vitamin D nutrition and bone disease of the elderly. *Public Health Nutrition* 4(2) (April): 547–59.

Griffin, S. O., K. Jones, and S. L. Tomar. 2001. An economic evaluation of community water fluoridation. *Journal of Public Health Dentistry* 61(2): 78–86.

Heaney, Mark L., Jeffrey R. Gardner, Nicos Karasavvas, David W. Golde, David A. Scheinberg, Emily A. Smith, and Owen A. O'Connor. 2008. Vitamin C Antagonizes the Cytotoxic Effects of Antineoplastic Drugs. *Cancer Research* 68, no. 19 (October 1): 8031-8038. doi:10.1158/0008-5472.CAN-08-1490.

Johnson, W. A. and G. L. Landry. 1998. Nutritional supplements: Fact vs. fiction. *Adolescent Medicine (Philadelphia, Pa.)* 9(3) (October): 501–513, vi.

Kessler, David. 2009. *The End of Overeating: Taking Control of the Insatiable North American Appetite.* Toronto: McClelland & Stewart.

Kurlansky, Mark. 2002. *Salt: A World History.* New York: Walker & Co.

National Institutes of Health. NIH state-of-the-science conference statement on multivitamin/mineral supplements and chronic disease prevention. 2006 *NIH Consensus and State-of-the-Science Statements* 23(2): 1–30.

Pauling, Linus Carl. 1995. *Vitamin C and the Common Cold.* Cutchogue, New York: Buccaneer Books.

CHAPTER 7.
ORIGINS: FOOD FOR THOUGHT

Eaton S. B., Melvin Konner, and Marjorie Shostak. 1988. Stone agers in the fast lane: Chronic degenerative diseases in evolutionary perspective. *The American Journal of Medicine* 84(4) (April): 739–49. doi: 10.1016/0002-9343(88)90113-1.

Eaton, S. Boyd and Stanley B. Eaton. 2003. An evolutionary perspective on human physical activity: Implications for health. *Comparative Biochemistry and Physiology. Part A, Molecular & Integrative Physiology* 136(1) (September): 153– 59.

Eaton, S. Boyd. 2006. The ancestral human diet: What was it and should it be a paradigm for contemporary nutrition? *Proceedings of the Nutrition Society* 65(1) (February): 1–6. doi: 10.1079/PNS2005471.

Richards, M. P. 2002. A brief review of the archaeological evidence for Palaeolithic and Neolithic subsistence. *European Journal of Clinical Nutrition* 56(12) (December): 16 p following 1,262. doi: 10.1038/sj.ejcn.1601646.

Starling, Anne P. and Jay T. Stock. 2007. Dental indicators of health and stress in early Egyptian and Nubian agriculturalists: A difficult transition and gradual recovery. *American Journal of Physical Anthropology* 134(4) (December): 520–28. doi: 10.1002/ajpa.20700.

CHAPTER 8.
DENTAL DECAY: THE PREVENTABLE SCOURGE

Beltrán-Aguilar, Eugenio D., Laurie K. Barker, María Teresa Canto, Bruce A. Dye, Barbara F. Gooch, Susan O. Griffin, Jeffrey Hyman, et al. 2005. Surveillance for dental caries, dental sealants, tooth retention, edentulism, and enamel fluorosis—United States, 1988–1994 and 1999–2002. *MMWR. Surveillance Summaries: Morbidity and Mortality Weekly Report. Surveillance Summaries / CDC* 54(3) (August 26): 1–43.

Cockburn, Thomas Aidan, Eve Cockburn, and Theodore A. Reyman. 1998. *Mummies, Disease and Ancient Cultures.* 2nd ed. Cambridge: Cambridge University Press: 28.

CHAPTER 9.
YOUR GUMS, YOUR HEART

Abou-Raya, Suzan, Amr Naeem, Kheir Hassan Abou-El, and Beltagy Sheriff El. 2002. Coronary artery disease and periodontal disease: Is there a link? *Angiology* 53(2): 141–48.

Beck, J. D., J. Pankow, H. A. Tyroler, and S. Offenbacher. 1999. Dental infections and atherosclerosis. *American Heart Journal* 138, no. 5 (November): S528-533.

Beevi, Leena, Shashikanth Hedge, Rajesh Kashyap, and Arun Kumar. 2009. Vaccines and periodontal diseases—An insight. *Dental Update* 36(10) (December): 635–38.

Cronin, Aaron. 2009. Periodontal disease is a risk marker for coronary heart disease? *Evidence-Based Dentistry* 10(1): 22. doi: 10.1038/sj.ebd.6400634.

Dykes, R. M., F. Grundy, and E. Lewis-Faning. 1953. Illness during the first five years of life; results of an inquiry in the borough of Luton. *British Journal of Preventive & Social Medicine* 7, no. 2 (April): 31–41.

Löe, H. 1967. The gingival index, the plaque index and the retention index systems. *Journal of Periodontology* 38(6) (December): Suppl: 610–16.

Mattila, K. J. 1993. Dental infections as a risk factor for acute myocardial infarction. *European Heart Journal* 14(Suppl K) (December): 51–53.

Oe, Yoko, Hirofumi Soejima, Hideki Nakayama, Takashi Fukunaga, Koichi Sugamura, Hiroaki Kawano, Seigo Sugiyama, et al. 2009. Significant association between score of periodontal disease and coronary artery disease. *Heart and Vessels* 24(2) (March): 103–07. doi: 10.1007/s00380-008-1096-z.

Thorburn, A. W., J. C. Brand, and A. S. Truswell. 1987. Slowly digested and absorbed carbohydrate in traditional bushfoods: a protective factor against diabetes? *The American Journal of Clinical Nutrition* 45, no. 1 (January): 98–106.

CHAPTER 10.
THE DEADLY QUARTET: EXCESS WEIGHT AND OBESITY

Cleave, Thomas. 1974. *The Saccharine Disease.* Bristol: John Wright and Sons Limited.

Cleave, T. L. 1975. The saccharine disease. *Transactions of the Medical Society of London* 91: 63–64.

Dedoussis, G. V. Z., A. C. Kaliora, and D. B. Panagiotakos. 2007. Genes, diet and type 2 diabetes mellitus: A review. *The Review of Diabetic Studies: RDS* 4(1): 13–24. doi:10.1900/RDS.2007.4.13.

Dykes, Robert M., Fred Grundy, and E. Lewis-Faning. 1953. Illness during the First Five Years of Life. *British Journal of Preventive & Social Medicine* 7, no. 2 (April): 31-42.

Flegal, Katherine M., Margaret D. Carroll, Cynthia L. Ogden, and Clifford L. Johnson. 2002. Prevalence and trends in obesity among US adults, 1999–2000. *JAMA: The Journal of the American Medical Association* 288(14) (October 9): 1723–27.

Grande, F., J. T. Anderson, C. Chlouverakis, M. Proja, and A. Keys. 1965. Effect of dietary cholesterol on man's serum lipids. *The Journal of Nutrition* 87(1) (September): 52–62.

Hujoel, P. 2009. Dietary carbohydrates and dental-systemic diseases. *Journal of Dental Research* 88(6) (June): 490–502. doi: 10.1177/0022034509337700.

Keys, A. 1965. Dietary survey methods in studies on cardiovascular epidemiology. *Voeding* 26 (July 15): 464–83.

Lubetkin, Erica I. and Haomiao Jia. 2009. Health-related quality of life, quality-adjusted life years, and quality-adjusted life expectancy in New York City from 1995 to 2006. *Journal of Urban Health: Bulletin of the New York Academy of Medicine* 86(4) (July): 551–61. doi: 10.1007/s11524-009-9344-9.

Onishi, Norimitsu. 2008. Japan, seeking trim waists, measures millions. *The New York Times* June 13, sec. International/Asia Pacific. http://www.nytimes.com/2008/06/13/world/asia/13fat.html?_r=1&scp=1&sq=metabo&st=cse.

Vancheri, F., A. Burgio, and R. Dovico. 2007. From "deadly quartet" to "metabolic syndrome": An analysis of its clinical relevance. *Recenti Progressi in Medicina* 98(3): 192–200.

Whitlock, Gary, Sarah Lewington, Paul Sherliker, Robert Clarke, Jonathan Emberson, Jim Halsey, Nawab Qizilbash, Rory Collins, and Richard Peto. 2009. Body-mass index and cause-specific mortality in 900,000 adults: collaborative analyses of 57 prospective studies. *Lancet* 373(9,669) (March 28): 1083–96. doi: 10.1016/S0140-6736(09)60318-4.

Yudkin, J. 1965. Evolution, history, and nutrition: their bearing on oral disease and other diseases of civilization. *The Dental Practitioner and Dental Record* 16(2) (October): 60–64.

Zahran, Hatice S., Rosemarie Kobau, David G. Moriarty, Matthew M. Zack, James Holt, and Ralph Donehoo. 2005. Health-related quality of life surveillance—United States, 1993–2002. *MMWR. Surveillance Summaries: Morbidity and Mortality Weekly Report. Surveillance Summaries / CDC* 54(4) (October 28): 1–35.

CHAPTER 11.
THE DEADLY QUARTET: ELEVATED BLOOD FATS

Bang, H. O., J. Dyerberg, and H. M. Sinclair. 1980. The composition of the Eskimo food in north western Greenland. *The American Journal of Clinical Nutrition* 33(12) (December): 2,657–61.

Bersamin, Andrea, Bret R. Luick, Irena B. King, Judith S. Stern, and Sheri Zidenberg-Cherr. 2008. Westernizing diets influence fat intake, red blood cell fatty acid composition, and health in remote Alaskan Native communities in the center for Alaska Native health study. *Journal of the American Dietetic*

Association 108(2) (February): 266–73. doi: 10.1016/j. jada.2007.10.046.

Bjerregaard, P., G. Mulvad, and H. S. Pedersen. 1997. Cardiovascular risk factors in Inuit of Greenland. *International Journal of Epidemiology* 26(6) (December): 1,182–90.

Dedoussis, G. V. Z., A. C. Kaliora, and D. B. Panagiotakos. 2007. Genes, diet and type 2 diabetes mellitus: A review. *The Review of Diabetic Studies: RDS* 4(1): 13–24. doi:10.1900/ RDS.2007.4.13.

Dyerberg, J., H. O. Bang, and N. Hjorne. 1975. Fatty acid composition of the plasma lipids in Greenland Eskimos. *The American Journal of Clinical Nutrition* 28(9) (September): 958–66.

Hofmann, Susanna M. and Matthias H. Tschöp. 2009. Dietary sugars: A fat difference. *The Journal of Clinical Investigation* 119(5) (May): 1,089–92.

Joseph, A., D. Ackerman, J. D. Talley, J. Johnstone, and J. Kupersmith. 1993. Manifestations of coronary atherosclerosis in young trauma victims—An autopsy study. *Journal of the American College of Cardiology* 22(2) (August): 459–67.

Luoma, P. V., S. Näyhä, K. Sikkilä, and J. Hassi. 1995. High serum alpha-tocopherol, albumin, selenium and cholesterol, and low mortality from coronary heart disease in northern Finland. *Journal of Internal Medicine* 237(1) (January): 49–54.

Perona, Javier S., María-Isabel Covas, Montserrat Fitó, Rosana Cabello-Moruno, Fernando Aros, Dolores Corella, Emilio Ros, et al. 2009. Reduction in systemic and VLDL triacylglycerol concentration after a 3-month Mediterranean-style diet in high-cardiovascular-risk subjects. *The Journal of Nutritional Biochemistry* (December 3). doi: 10.1016/j.

jnutbio.2009.07.005. http://www.ncbi.nlm.nih.gov/pubmed /19962297.

Sharma, Sangita, Xia Cao, Cindy Roache, Annie Buchan, Rhonda Reid, and Joel Gittelsohn. 2010. Assessing dietary intake in a population undergoing a rapid transition in diet and lifestyle: The Arctic Inuit in Nunavut, Canada. *The British Journal of Nutrition* 103(5) (March): 749–59. doi:10.1017/ S0007114509992224.

CHAPTER 12.
THE DEADLY QUARTET: DIABETES

Dedoussis, George V. Z., Andriana C. Kaliora, and Demosthenes B. Panagiotakos. 2007. Genes, diet and type 2 diabetes mellitus: A review. *The Review of Diabetic Studies: RDS* 4(1): 13–24. doi: 10.1900/RDS.2007.4.13.

Gross, Lee S., Li Li, Earl S. Ford, and Simin Liu. 2004. Increased consumption of refined carbohydrates and the epidemic of type 2 diabetes in the United States: An ecologic assessment. *The American Journal of Clinical Nutrition* 79(5) (May): 774–79.

Kopp, Wolfgang. 2003. High-insulinogenic nutrition—An etiologic factor for obesity and the metabolic syndrome? *Metabolism: Clinical and Experimental* 52(7) (July): 840–44.

McKeown, Pascal P., Karen Logan, Michelle C. McKinley, Ian S. Young, and Jayne V. Woodside. 2010. Session 4: CVD, diabetes and cancer: Evidence for the use of the Mediterranean diet in patients with CHD. *The Proceedings of the Nutrition Society* 69(1) (February): 45–60. doi: 10.1017/ S0029665109991856.

Murtaugh, Maureen A., David R. Jacobs, Brenda Jacob, Lyn M. Steffen, and Leonard Marquart. 2003. Epidemiological support for the protection of whole grains against diabetes. *The Proceedings of the Nutrition Society* 62(1) (February): 143–49.

Tabatabai, A. and S. Li. 2000. Dietary fiber and type 2 diabetes. *Clinical Excellence for Nurse Practitioners: The International Journal of NPACE* 4(5) (September): 272–76.

Tekavec, Carol. 2009. Systemic diseases and dental treatment: talking with your patients. *Dentistry Today* 28(6) (June): 108–109.

Thorburn, A W, J C Brand, K O'Dea, R M Spargo, and A S Truswell. 1987. Plasma glucose and insulin responses to starchy foods in Australian aborigines: a population now at high risk of diabetes. *The American Journal of Clinical Nutrition* 46, no. 2 (August): 282-285.

Vancheri, Federico, Antonio Burgio, and Rossana Dovico. 2007. From "deadly quartet" to "metabolic syndrome": An analysis of its clinical relevance. *Recenti Progressi in Medicina* 98(3) (March): 192–200.

Venn, B. J., and J. I. Mann. 2004. Cereal grains, legumes and diabetes. *European Journal of Clinical Nutrition* 58(11) (November): 1443–61. doi: 10.1038/sj.ejcn.1601995.

CHAPTER 13.
THE DEADLY QUARTET: HYPERTENSION AND HEART DISEASE

Anderson, J. W., T. J. Hanna, X. Peng, and R. J. Kryscio. 2000. Whole grain foods and heart disease risk. *Journal of the American College of Nutrition* 19(3) (June): 291S–299S.

Abu-Saad, K., S. Weitzman, Y. Abu-Rabiah, H. Abu-Shareb, and D. Fraser. Rapid lifestyle, diet and health changes among urban Bedouin Arabs of southern Israel. Food, nutrition and agriculture – 2001. Food and Agriculture Organization of the United Nations. http://www.fao.org/docrep/003/y0600m/y0600m06.htm#TopOfPage.

Benson, Herbert. 1983. The relaxation response: Its subjective and objective historical precedents and physiology. *Trends in Neurosciences* 6: 281–84. doi: 10.1016/0166-2236(83)90120-0.

Eaton, S. Boyd. 2006. The ancestral human diet: What was it and should it be a paradigm for contemporary nutrition? *Proceedings of the Nutrition Society* 65(1) (February): 1–6. doi: 10.1079/PNS2005471.

Hu, Frank B., Eric B. Rimm, Meir J. Stampfer, Alberto Ascherio, Donna Spiegelman, and Walter C. Willett. 2000. Prospective study of major dietary patterns and risk of coronary heart disease in men. *American Journal of Clinical Nutrition* 72(4) (October 1): 912–21.

Kitamura, Kazuya, Michael Fetters, Kiyoshi Sano, Juichi Sato, and Nobutaro Ban. 2009. Lifestyle changes of Japanese people on overseas assignment in Michigan, USA. *Asia Pacific Family Medicine* 8(1): 7. doi: 10.1186/1447-056X-8-7.

Kopp, Wolfgang. 2003. High-insulinogenic nutrition—An etiologic factor for obesity and the metabolic syndrome? *Metabolism: Clinical and Experimental* 52(7) (July): 840–44.

McKeown, Pascal P., Karen Logan, Michelle C. McKinley, Ian S. Young, and Jayne V. Woodside. 2009. Session 4: CVD, diabetes and cancer: Evidence for the use of the Mediterranean diet in patients with CHD. *The Proceedings of the Nutrition Society* (December 15): 1–16. doi: 10.1017/S0029665109991856.

Ness, A. R., and J. W. Powles. 1997. Fruit and vegetables, and cardiovascular disease: A review. *International Journal of Epidemiology.* 26(1) (February 1): 1–13. doi: 10.1093/ije/26.1.1.

O'Dea, K., R. M. Spargo, and P. J. Nestel. 1982. Impact of westernization on carbohydrate and lipid metabolism in Australian Aborigines. *Diabetologia* 22(3) (March 1): 148–53. doi: 10.1007/BF00283742.

Pavan, Lucia; Edoardo Casiglia, Laura M. Braga, Carvalho, Mikolaj Winnicki, Massimo Puato, Paolo Pauletto, and Achille C. Pessina. 1999. Effects of a traditional lifestyle on the cardiovascular risk profile: The Amondava population of the Brazilian Amazon. Comparison with matched African, Italian and Polish populations. *Journal of Hypertension*: June 1999 17(6): 749–56.

Vorster, H. H. 2002. The emergence of cardiovascular disease during urbanisation of Africans. *Public Health Nutrition* 5(1) (February): 239–43.

CHAPTER 14.
CONSTIPATION AND ITS CONSEQUENCES: VARICOSE VEINS,
VARICOCELE, HEMORRHOIDS, DEEP VENOUS THROMBOSIS,
DIVERTICULITIS, AND YES, EXCESS WEIGHT

Bahadursingh, Anil M., Kathy S. Virgo, Donald L. Kaminski, and Walter E. Longo. 2003. Spectrum of disease and outcome of complicated diverticular disease. *American Journal of Surgery* 186(6) (December): 696–701.

Beebe-Dimmer, Jennifer L., John R. Pfeifer, Jennifer S. Engle, and David Schottenfeld. 2005. The epidemiology of chronic venous insufficiency and varicose veins. *Annals of*

Epidemiology 15, no. 3 (March): 175–184. doi:10.1016/j. annepidem.2004.05.015.

Biyani, Chandra Shekhar, Jon Cartledge, and Günter Janetschek. 2009. Varicocele. *Clinical Evidence.* http://www.ncbi.nlm. nih.gov/pubmed/19445764.

Burkitt, D. P. 1976. Varicose veins: Facts and fantasy. *Archives of Surgery (Chicago, Ill.: 1960)* 111(12) (December): 1327–32.

Cherbut, C., A. C. Aube, N. Mekki, C. Dubois, D. Lairon, and J. L. Barry. 1997. Digestive and metabolic effects of potato and maize fibres in human subjects. *The British Journal of Nutrition* 77(1) (January): 33–46.

Cleave, Thomas. 1974 *The Saccharine Disease.* Bristol: John Wright and Sons Limited.

Esmon, Charles T. 2009. Basic mechanisms and pathogenesis of venous thrombosis. *Blood Reviews* 23(5) (September): 225–29. doi: 10.1016/j.blre.2009.07.002.

Evers, Johannes, L. H. Hans, John Collins, and Jane Clarke. 2009. Surgery or embolisation for varicoceles in subfertile men. *Cochrane Database of Systematic Reviews (Online)* 1: CD000479. doi: 10.1002/14651858.CD000479.pub4.

Floch, Martin H, and Iona Bina. 2004. The natural history of diverticulitis: fact and theory. *Journal of Clinical Gastroenterology* 38, no. 5 (June): S2-7.

Haas, Peter, Thomas Fox, and Gabriel Haas. 1984. The pathogenesis of hemorrhoids. *Diseases of the Colon & Rectum* 27(7) (July 1): 442–50. doi: 10.1007/BF02555533.

Hoffmann, R. M., and W. Kruis. 2005. Diverticulosis and diverticulitis. *Der Internist* 46(6) (June): 671–83; quiz 684. doi: 10.1007/s00108-005-1403-z.

Hovey, Amynta L., Gwyn P. Jones, Helen M. Devereux, and Karen Z. Walker. 2003. Whole cereal and legume seeds increase faecal short chain fatty acids compared to ground seeds. *Asia Pacific Journal of Clinical Nutrition* 12(4): 477–82.

Nabi, G., S. Asterlings, D. R. Greene, and R. L. Marsh. 2004. Percutaneous embolization of varicoceles: Outcomes and correlation of semen improvement with pregnancy. *Urology* 63(2) (February): 359–63. doi: 10.1016/j. urology.2003.09.026.

Parra-Blanco, Adolfo. 2006. Colonic diverticular disease: Pathophysiology and clinical picture. *Digestion* 73(Suppl 1): 47–57. doi: 10.1159/000089779.

Pfeifer, J. 2008. Diverticulitis. *Acta Chirurgica Iugoslavica* 55(3): 97–102.

Robertson, L., C. Evans, and F. G. R. Fowkes. 2008. Epidemiology of chronic venous disease. *Phlebology / Venous Forum of the Royal Society of Medicine* 23(3): 103–111. doi: 10.1258/ phleb.2007.007061.

Soffer, Y., R. Ron-El, J. Sayfan, and E. Caspi. 1983. Spermatic vein ligation in varicocele: prognosis and associated male and female infertility factors. *Fertility and Sterility* 40(3) (September): 353–57.

Spencer, Frederick, Cathy Emery, Samuel Joffe, Luigi Pacifico, Darleen Lessard, George Reed, Joel Gore, and Robert Goldberg. 2009. Incidence rates, clinical profile, and outcomes of patients with venous thromboembolism. The Worcester VTE study. *Journal of Thrombosis and Thrombolysis* (July 24). doi: 10.1007/s11239-009-0378-3. http://www. ncbi.nlm.nih.gov/pubmed/19629642.

Spencer, Frederick A., Cathy Emery, Darleen Lessard, Frederick Anderson, Sri Emani, Jayashri Aragam, Richard C. Becker, and Robert J. Goldberg. 2006. The Worcester Venous

Thromboembolism study: A population-based study of the clinical epidemiology of venous thromboembolism. *Journal of General Internal Medicine* 21(7) (July): 722–27. doi: 10.1111/j.1525-1497.2006.00458.x.

Spinzi, Giancarlo, Arnaldo Amato, Gianni Imperiali, Nicoletta Lenoci, Giovanna Mandelli, Silvia Paggi, Franco Radaelli, Natalia Terreni, and Vittorio Terruzzi. 2009. Constipation in the elderly: Management strategies. *Drugs & Aging* 26(6): 469–74. doi: 10.2165/00002512-200926060-00003.

Sudoł-Szopińska, Iwona, Krzysztof Błachowiak, and Piotr Koziński. 2006. [Influence of environmental risk factors on the development of chronic vein insufficiency]. *Medycyna Pracy* 57(4): 365–73.

Traber, J., L. Mazzolai, and S. Läuchli. 2009. [Epidemiology of chronic venous insufficiency--Swiss survey with surprising results]. *Praxis* 98(14) (July 8): 749–55. doi: 10.1024/1661-8157.98.14.749.

Trepel, Friedrich. 2004. [Dietary fibre: more than a matter of dietetics. I. Compounds, properties, physiological effects]. *Wiener Klinische Wochenschrift* 116(14) (July 31): 465–76.

Vuksan, Vladimir, Alexandra L. Jenkins, David J. A. Jenkins, Alexander L. Rogovik, John L. Sievenpiper, and Elena Jovanovski. 2008. Using cereal to increase dietary fiber intake to the recommended level and the effect of fiber on bowel function in healthy persons consuming North American diets. *The American Journal of Clinical Nutrition* 88(5) (November): 1256–62.

Winterhalder, B., R. Larsen, and R. B. Thomas. 1974. Dung as an essential resource in a highland Peruvian community *Human Ecology.* 2(2): 89–104.

CHAPTER 15.
THE ONLY GUIDE TO EATING YOU'LL EVER NEED

Blumenschine, Robert J., Henry T. Bunn, Valerius Geist, Fumiko Ikawa-Smith, Curtis W. Marean, Anthony G. Payne, John Tooby, and Nikolaas J. van der Merwe. 1987. Characteristics of an early hominid scavenging niche [and Comments and Reply]. *Current Anthropology* 28(4) (October): 383–407.

Foster, Gary D., Holly R. Wyatt, James O. Hill, Brian G. McGuckin, Carrie Brill, B. Selma Mohammed, Philippe O. Szapary, Daniel J. Rader, Joel S. Edman, and Samuel Klein. 2003. A Randomized Trial of a Low-Carbohydrate Diet for Obesity. *North England Journal of Medicine* 348(21) (May 22): 2,082–90. doi: 10.1056/NEJMoa022207.

Fry, William E., and Stephen B. Goodwin. 1997. Resurgence of the Irish Potato Famine Fungus. *BioScience* 47(6) (June): 363–71.

Hodge, W. 1951. Three native tuber foods of the high Andes. *Economic Botany* 5(2) (April 1): 185–201. doi: 10.1007/BF02984776.

Kessler, David. 2009. *The End of Overeating: Taking Control of the Insatiable North American Appetite.* Toronto: McClelland & Stewart.

Keys, A., A. Menotti, M. J. Karvonen, C. Aravanis, H. Blackburn, R. Buzina, B. S. Djordjevic, A. S. Dontas, F. Fidanza, and M. H. Keys. 1986. The diet and 15-year death rate in the seven countries study. *American Journal of Epidemiology* 124, no. 6 (December): 903–915.

Serdula, Mary K., Ali H. Mokdad, David F. Williamson, Deborah A. Galuska, James M. Mendlein, and Gregory W. Heath. 1999. Prevalence of Attempting Weight Loss and Strategies for Controlling Weight. *JAMA* 282(14) (October 13): 1,353–58. doi: 10.1001/jama.282.14.1353.

CONCLUSION

American Cancer Society. 2000. California lung cancer rates drop significantly. *ACS News Center.* http://www.cancer.org/docroot/NWS/content/NWS_1_1x_California_Lung_Cancer_Rates_Drop_Significantly_.asp.

Polednak, A. P. 2008. Tobacco control indicators and lung cancer rates in young adults by state in the United States. *Tobacco Control* 17(1) (February): 66–69. doi: 10.1136/tc.2007.020925.

Smith, R. A., and T. J. Glynn. 2000. Epidemiology of lung cancer. *Radiologic Clinics of North America* 38(3) (May): 453–70.

Temple, N. J., and D. P. Burkitt. 1993. Towards a new system of health: The challenge of Western disease. *Journal of Community Health* 18(1) (February): 37–47.

Index

Page numbers with "*n*" refer to footnotes
Page number in **Bold** refer to References section in back of book

diets
  Atkins, 97
  balanced, 16n6, 33
  Biggest Loser Diet, 92
  Bob Greene best life, 92
  Body for Life, 97
  Cabbage Soup, 100
  Cheater's Diet, 100
  Cookie Diet, 100
  Dr. Phil's Ultimate Weight
      Solution diet,
      92–93
  Eat Right for Your Blood
      Type, 101
  Eat This, Not That, 98
  French Women Don't Get Fat,
      98–99
  Fruit Flush, 101
  Glycemic Index Diet (Low
      Glycemic Diet), 93
  health issues relating to, xvi
  high-protein diets, 97
  Jenny Craig Weight Loss
      Program, 93
  lifespan and, 21
  Macrobiotic Diet, 102
  Martha's Vineyard Diet
      Detox, 102
  "Mayo Clinic," 102–103
  Mayo Clinic Diet, 94
  Medifest Diet Plan, 94
  Mediterranean Diet, 72,
      94–95, 100, 102,
      104
  Morning Banana Diet, 103
  New Beverly Hills Diet, 103
  NutriSystem Diet, 95
  nutrition and, 4
  Okinawa Diet, 95–96
  The 100-Mile Diet, 101–
      102
  Organic Food Diets, 103
  Paleolithic (Old Stone Age)
      Diet, 104
  Pritikin Principle, 99
  Raw Food Diet, 98
  "see food," 40
  Slim-Fast Weight Loss Plan,
      96
  South Beach, 93
  vegetarian and vegan
      lifestyle, 97–98
  water in, 27
  Weight Watchers, 96
  weight-loss (*See* weight-loss
      diets)
  Weil's Diet (Dr. Andrew),
      96
  You: On a Diet, 96–97
  Zone, 93
  The Zone Diet, 99
diffuse/concentrated
      phenomenon, 11–13
diseases. *See also individual
      diseases*
  cause of, 58–59n18
  causes of (*See* chronic
      diseases)
  conditions of lifestyle, xvii
  emergence of chronic, 7
diseases of civilization
  causes of, 47, 48

Okamura, Tomonori, 21, **112**
O'Keefe, James H., **107,** xvi
Okinawa Diet, 95–96
olive oil, 20
Omega-3 fatty acids, 19, 64
Omega-6 fatty acids, 19
The 100-Mile Diet, 101–102
Onishi, Norimitsu, 59, **119**
Oparin, Alexander, 22*n*7
organic food, real food *vs.,* 6
origins of human beings, 37–41, 37*n*14
"-ose" suffix in ingredients, 13, 26, xviii
overeating, impulsive, 92–93

P

Pacifico, Luigi, 80, **127**
Paggi, Silvia, 77, **128**
Paleolithic (Old Stone Age) Diet, 104
Panagiotakos, Demosthenes B., 58, **119, 121–122**
pancreas, 65, 66
Pankow, J., 53, **117**
Papas, A. S., 26, **113**
Parker, David M., 16, **110**
Parra-Blanco, Adolfo, 80, **127**
Pauletto, Paolo, 70, **125**
Pauling, Linus Carl, 31, 31*n*9, **116**
Pavan, Lucia, 70, **125**
Payne, Anthony G., 98, **129**
pectin, 29, 75–76
Pedersen, H. S., 64, **121**
Peng, X., 70, **123**

periodontitis, 51, 52, 53. *See also* gums
Perona, Javier S., 63, **121**
Perrin, Anne-Elisabeth, 24, 28, **113**
Pessina, Achille C., 70, **125**
Peto, Richard, 57, **120**
Pfeifer
  J., **127**
  John R., **125**
Pfeifer, J., 80, **127**
Pfeifer, John R., 78, **125**
physical activity, chronic diseases and, 7
pit and fissure sealants, application of, 47
plant proteins, 16
plums, diffuse/concentrated continuing of, 12–13
Polednak, A. P., 105, **130**
polyunsaturated, 19
Popkin, B. M., 23, **113**
Poplove, M., 34, **114**
population size, food and, 6
Portion Control method, 88–89
potatoes, 9, 67, 84–85
Powles, J. W., 72, **125**
prayer, 73
prevalence, definition of, 39, 39*n*15
primordial soup of molecules, 22, 22*n*7
Pritikin Longevity Center (Miami), 99
processed foods, 10–11, 50, 72

increase usage of sugar and
rise in, 13
as predictor of colonic stasis,
76
as predictor of diverticulitis,
81
as predictor of elevated
blood fats, 63
preventing, 45–48
proteins that prevent, 16
reductions in, 47
refined carbohydrates and,
46
water and, 25–26
tooth enamel, 34
toothpastes, 26, 47
Traber, J., 78, **128**
trans fats, 19, 20, 21
Treacy, B., 31, **115**
Trepel, Friedrich., **128**
Truswell, A. S., 67, **118, 123**
Tschöp, H, 63, **121**
Tyroler, H. A., 53, **117**

U

Ultimate Weight Solution diet,
Dr. Phil's, 92–93
United States government
food guides, 35, 35n13
health websites, 27n8,
89–90
recommended daily water
intake, 24
unsaturated fats, 19
Urine, 24

U.S. Food and Drug
Administration, 27n8

V

van der Merve, Nikolaas J., 98,
129
van Duijn, G., **112**
van Staveren, Wija A., 24, 28,
113
Vancheri, Federico, 55, **120,
123**
varicocele
about, 78–79
abuse of foods and, 10
in ancient human beings,
47
cause of, xvii
constipation and, 87
increase usage of sugar and
rise in, 13
varicose veins
about, 77–78
abuse of foods and, 10
in ancient human beings,
47
cause of, xvii
constipation and, 87
increase usage of sugar and
rise in, 13
vegetable oils, 20, 72, 85, 92
vegetables
as carbohydrates, 9
fresh, 15
proteins in, 16
sugar in, 13
water in, 24